HERBAL CURES
HEALING REMEDIES FROM IRELAND

GW00536254

HERBAL CURES

HEALING REMEDIES FROM IRELAND

CHRISTINE SCALLAN

Newleaf

Newleaf
an imprint of
Gill & Macmillan Ltd
Hume Avenue, Park West, Dublin 12
with associated companies throughout the world
www.gillmacmillan.ie
© Christine Scallan 1994, 2003
First published in 1994 under the title *Irish Herbal Cures*
This edition first published 2003
0 7171 3623 X

Design and print origination by
O'K Graphic Design, Dublin

Illustrations by Fiona Fewer

Printed in Malaysia

The paper used in this book is made from the wood pulp of managed forests. For every tree felled, at least one tree is planted, thereby renewing natural resources.

A catalogue record is available for this book from the British Library.

1 3 5 4 2

The information contained in this book is in no way intended to replace professional medical advice and treatment. If you are in any doubt about your health or if you are pregnant, always consult your doctor.

Contents

CONTENTS

PART II AILMENTS   97

CONTENTS

Glossary

Compress
A compress is a pad of gauze or lint soaked in an infusion or decoction and bandaged to the skin. It can be either warm or cold.

Decoction
A decoction is made by soaking herbs in cold water for a short while, then bringing them gently to the boil and simmering for twenty minutes. Use at the rate of one tablespoonful of the dried herb to 1.1 litres (2 pints) of water. Decoctions are most often applied externally. Soups and stews are a type of decoction and you will know from your own experience that, when flavouring them with herbs, a little goes a long way.

Herbal oil
Fill a clear jar or bottle with freshly picked herbs and immerse them in safflower or sunflower oil. Cover the jar with muslin and place on a sunny windowsill or some other warm place. Steep for two weeks, shaking daily. Strain, bottle and label.

Infusion
The words tisane, infusion and tea are used interchangeably. A tisane is made by pouring approximately 300 ml (½ pint) of hot water over one teaspoonful of the dried herb (or two teaspoonfuls of the fresh herb). Allow to infuse for five minutes, strain and use. Most of the tisanes mentioned in this book are readily available in health food shops as tea-bags. Wherever mixtures are given as the basis of a tisane they can usually be purchased already mixed at health food shops. If they are not accessible in this form, discuss their proportions with a herbalist. Where not otherwise stated, the usual dose of an infusion is one wineglassful per day.

Ointments, creams and unguents

Mix 30 g (1 oz) of beeswax, lanolin or lard with 115 ml (4 fl oz) of herbal oil. Simmer gently for ten minutes, constantly stirring the mixture. Strain through muslin into a container with a wide top. Cover and label.

Poultices and fomentations

A poultice is a medicinal substance which is warm and pasty, held between two layers of muslin and applied to the skin. It is removed when it cools.

Syrup

Mix three tablespoonfuls of honey (sugar will do but is not as good and will not last as long) in 300 ml (½ pint) of an infusion of the appropriate herb. Bring slowly to the boil, stirring until the mixture thickens to a syrup. Allow to cool and pour into a clean glass bottle. Cover and preserve in the refrigerator.

Tincture

A tincture is made by leaving either a fresh or a dried herb to steep in a solvent, most often alcohol or occasionally alcohol with some water added. The proportions are generally five parts of alcohol (vodka is most commonly used) to one part of crushed herb. Put the crushed herb into a glass bottle or jar and pour on the vodka. Put the stopper in the bottle and leave it for one week, then strain and squeeze out the residue. Where possible, do not pick herbs in areas that have been chemically polluted.

Herbs are best when picked in full sunshine and dried quickly away from the sunlight. Exceptions to this rule will be indicated in the text.

Only stainless steel or Pyrex containers should be used for heating herbs.

Introduction

O the greater fleabane that grew at the back of the potato pit:
I often trampled through it looking for rabbit burrows!
The burnet saxifrage was there in profusion
And the autumn gentian —
I knew them all by eyesight long before I knew their names.
We were in love before we were introduced.

In his poem 'On reading a book on common wild flowers', Patrick Kavanagh expressed a feeling many of us will have experienced: 'I knew them all by eyesight long before I knew their names. We were in love before we were introduced.' This book will not even attempt to introduce 'them all'. My aim rather is to stay close to the earth; to take a stroll through the fields and woods, the highways and byways; to encounter the familiar and some of the less familiar herbs of our countryside; and to become better acquainted with these loveliest and most useful of the friends of man.

'Science' we shall leave to the scientist, with the reminder that human beings and herbs had evolved in harmony for millions of years before science turned its attention to nature's laboratory. Great indeed are the achievements of science, particularly of medical science, in making use of herbs and plants for the benefit of human health. However, all is done by courtesy of nature, and impatience with nature has given us iatrogenic or 'doctor-caused' disease, an increasingly serious phenomenon. This is not to create a false opposition between doctor and herbalist — both pursue the rectification of health problems by the judicious application of refined herbal remedies. But perhaps we have all been at fault in the past in drawing a division between herbs as employed strictly for the restoration of health and herbs as part of everyday diet.

This book is written in the belief that the constant use of herbs, both as food and as flavouring, is related in many subtle ways to the general state of our health. It does not discuss specific herbal reme-dies in isolation from the broader context of our overall diet. The value of herbal 'cures' — whether self-administered, administered in their simpler forms by a herbalist or in their more sophisticated forms by a medical doctor — is, of course, taken into account; but only as part of a more comprehensive relationship with herbs. This relationship embraces a lore which extends back into prehistory and across the wide spaces of the world, and an instinct that is as old as the human race itself.

This book should not be considered in any way a substitute for a visit to your doctor. For although it is true that we no more receive all our healing from the hands of the medical profession than that we acquire all our education within the walls of schools and colleges, it must be emphasised that neither this book nor any other can take the place of a proper professional diagnosis. The circumstances and conditions of an illness will vary from person to person, and the ele-ments of treatment required are matters for the judgment of the practitioner treating that case. The question of the application of particular herbal, or any other, cures to individual cases lies quite outside the scope of this book. Rather, the perspective is best defined by Hippocrates' advice: 'Let your medicine be your food and your food your medicine.' The line between herbs taken for purely medicinal purposes and herbs taken as health-giving foods is difficult to determine, sometimes non-existent. Many of the herbal 'cures' discussed are in the nature of healthy additions to diet which can remedy illnesses or even prevent them from occurring. This latter they achieve by countering tendencies towards certain weak-nesses or by strengthening the overall health of the body, enabling it to overcome local difficulties.

It is also well to understand that, while one of the advantages of herbal preparations is that they rarely have the side-effects of con-ventional 'drug' treatments, herbs do interact with conventional drugs. For this reason, if you are being treated by a medical practi-tioner for a particular ailment, you should acquaint him or her with details of any herbal preparations you are taking and seek advice on whether or not to continue with them.

The book is divided into two main parts. Part I provides mono-graphs of a number of herbs with information on their therapeutic uses and some recipes. The herbs are chosen for their availability and the recipes for their practical character and the ready accessibil-ity of their ingredients. Part II considers some common ailments and some of the herbal 'cures' which have been applied to them, both professionally and popularly. Again the all-important matter of diet is kept in view.

The special health foods, honey, pollen, kelp, and apple cider vinegar, are discussed in an opening chapter. No powers of healing are claimed for any herb or health food beyond what is fairly widely agreed and the maxim 'A little goes a long way' is commended to your attention at all times.

Many of the herbal cures described in this book are used in more than one country and are of such antiquity that their origins are irretrievably lost. I call the book *Herbal Cures: Healing Remedies from Ireland* because most, if not all, of the cures described have been used and are being used in Ireland, from time to time and from place to place.

Food for Healthy Living

HONEY

The first thing to be said about honey is that only the bees can make it. Clever people have tried and failed. They have created synthetically all the substances to which honey can be scientifically reduced, combined those substances and found them to be exactly the same weight as the combined weight of similar amounts of their equivalents in real honey. But it hasn't worked. It has not provided the benefits of real honey. The secret of the bees remains undiscovered.

These efforts to outsmart nature have, however, furnished us with a great deal of knowledge about honey. We know that it contains natural sugars, proteins and mineral salts. We know that it differs according to its place of origin. The climate, the weather, the kinds of vegetation from which the bees draw the nectar and pollen, even the types of minerals in the soil: all play a part in determining the taste and composition of honey.

The first benefit which honey bestows is energy. Carbohydrate, the main requirement of tired muscle, is supplied by honey, which has the advantage of passing into the bloodstream with minimal expenditure of scarce energy. If you are fatigued and fed up try a small quantity of honey. More can, of course, be taken with very little danger as honey is the most benign of food substances; but large amounts belong more to curing alcoholic hangovers than to coping with general tiredness. If you take too much at one time you may lose your taste for it.

There is no better food for young children or for elderly people than honey. It is palatable, it is very easily digested and it encourages proper movement of the bowels. Honey is also of substantial benefit to those with weak hearts. Joggers might note that, as well as providing instant energy, honey helps to tone up the immune system, which is seriously weakened by exercise, leaving the body open to infective invasions which would otherwise be repulsed. Innumerable examples from the history of great achievers could be cited in support of honey as a source of physical energy and health. The success of Edmund Hillary, one of the first men to climb Mount Everest, has been attributed to the fact that he was a bee farmer in New Zealand.

Honey proves the wisdom of the principle, 'Let your medicine be your food and your food your medicine'. It has splendid antiseptic qualities; it halts the growth of germs and kills bacteria; it stimulates the heart and has a tonic effect on the entire system.

A substance called ceromel has for centuries past been used to cure ulcers in India. It is made up of four parts of honey to one part of beeswax. If you are preparing this remedy be sure to use soft and fairly new wax; the older wax gets hard, inflexible and practically impossible to digest, owing, it is said, to the constant traffic to and fro of the bees. I have met a man whose stomach was so badly ulcerated in his youth that doctors gave him up for lost. On the advice of a wise old lady he took honey in warm milk over a period of time. He is now a healthy octogenarian living happily with his second wife.

Honey as an inhalant in cases of asthma and bronchitis is seriously undervalued or not known of at all. A jar of honey held under the nose and inhaled will greatly help towards easing the breathing and restoring its normal rhythm. It is hard to know exactly why such inhalation is quite so helpful; scientific opinion links it to a combination of ethereal oils and various forms of alcohol in the honey. If you can get honey from coniferous forests you will have the very best of inhalants. A walk through a pine forest will be known to most people as a highly invigorating tonic for the lungs and respiratory system in general, and bees seem to bring together the turpentines and balsams from the conifers in a healing combination.

Many believe that the phenomenal healing powers of honey are due, at least in part, to its being hygroscopic: i.e. attracting and absorbing moisture. To this is attributed its ability to kill germs which must have moisture to live, which makes honey a first-class dressing for external wounds (including burns) and also for internal ailments such as ulcers. Honey is essential to sufferers from anaemia, helping to maintain the proper balance between haemoglobin and red corpuscles.

People who take alcoholic spirits to stimulate the action of the heart might consider the superiority of honey for this purpose. Whereas alcohol stimulates but does not provide a continuing source of energy, honey does both, gently and naturally. Spirits can have unpleasant and, cumulatively, serious after-effects; honey leaves no debt to be paid by the system. A teaspoonful of honey in a glass of water may not have the same immediate appeal to the seasoned spirits drinker as a glass of whiskey or brandy, but it will be more effective and will, given time, be just as palatable, if not indeed pleasantly habit-forming.

Honey has recently been discovered to help those whose blood lacks the essential clotting agents and who therefore tend to bleed unduly either externally or internally when cut or bruised. Vitamin K is the coagulation factor and the indications are that honey supplies this or some mysterious equivalent, and seems to supply it only where required. If these findings are eventually proven scientifically, they will only provide further evidence for what devotees of honey have long known: that honey is a marvellous agent of balance, fulfilling our particular needs at the right times and in the right amounts.

Honey has a special role to play in restoring the body gently in cases of malnutrition. It would be of inestimable value if peoples of Third World countries were taught the most advanced bee-management skills as, very often, those countries have massive sources of honey waiting to be harvested. Children suffering from malnutrition could probably be most easily brought back to normal health and bodyweight with the assistance of liberal amounts of honey. Diarrhoea, rickets and scurvy are only some of the accompaniments of malnutrition to be relieved by honey. Even in our comparatively well-fed Western nations there are more cases of malnutrition than might be immediately evident. People on a good diet can sometimes, for various reasons, be failing to absorb their nutritional requirements. Honey can make up the shortfall, partly because of its ready digestibility.

It is not possible to list the ailments for which honey will work its quiet wonders, but one worth a passing mention is rheumatism. Ancestral wisdom has it that bee-stings contain a cure for rheumatism. The general method of applying this cure is to confine about half a dozen bees in a matchbox, shake the box well in order to make them angry, and open it slowly over the rheumatic area making sure the bees don't escape. The rest of the process can safely be left to the bees. The sufferer may, of course, be allergic to bee-stings — or, more likely, allergic even to the thought of such a drastic and painful 'remedy', feeling that the cure might be worse than the disease. Take heart, it has been known for over fifty years that honey contains the same neutralising acids with which the stings effect their cure, and that taken internally it can be equally beneficial in cases of muscle atrophy and rheumatism. Beeswax, which is really honey with an enzyme added, has a marvellously curative effect when heated and put on the feet and hands of arthritis sufferers. Heat the wax carefully, never exposing it to naked flame. Put it in a container, immerse in a pot of water and simmer gently. This will both melt the wax and warm it to a bearable level, safely.

Where possible, honey should be bought directly from the beekeeper, because before being put on public sale it has usually been strained, in the process losing many of the additional 'goodies' — including pollen, wax, royal jelly and propolis.

Honey as Food

The value of honey in cooking has been appreciated for as long as records have been kept. The ancient Egyptians noted some of its uses. These days there are entire books of recipes for cooking with honey. I will confine myself to a few simple recipes, with the general note that there is hardly a dish of any kind to which honey would not make a delicious and nutritious contribution.

Honey cakes

Mix a cup of wheat or oat flakes, one tablespoonful of milk and one tablespoonful of honey. Do not bake but simply shape in small cakes and serve with stewed fruit. While you eat these delicious cakes remember that the Promised Land was a land overflowing with milk and honey.

Muesli

Soak a tablespoonful of flaked oatmeal in three tablespoonfuls of water for twelve hours, then mix with one tablespoonful of ground almonds, one tablespoonful of honey and a grated apple. Add a few chopped nuts and eat with yoghurt.

Honey dessert

Mix together a generous amount of honey and some finely chopped nuts. When thick, add some chopped fruit. Serve with yoghurt or cream.

Honey fudge
Put 225 g (½ lb) each of honey and of raw cane sugar, 55 g (2 oz) of butter and 150 ml (¼ pint) of milk in a saucepan. Heat gently, stirring all the time, until the sugar has dissolved. Add a pinch of cream of tartar and boil until it thickens. Remove from the heat, add a few drops of vanilla essence and beat well until thick and creamy. Pour into greased tins, mark into squares and allow to harden.

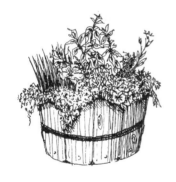

POLLEN —
the perfect food

Pollen is a fine granular substance which is released by the anther of the male flower to fertilise the ovule or germ cell of the female flower. It corresponds roughly to sperm in the animal world. Like honey it is amazingly complex in the range of its contents. It contains a spectrum of amino acids, which are the basis of proteins, the builders of muscles in our bodies. Collections of vitamins are also found in pollen, and minerals present include potassium, magnesium, calcium, iron, copper, zinc and silica. There are enzymes galore as well. The pollen grain itself, frequently extremely small, is also extremely tough — so tough that it is sometimes found intact in the geological strata which go back to when plants first began to grow on the earth. The worker bees feed the young bees on pollen and the queen bee will not start to lay eggs until she sees the pollen being brought into the hive in spring. If you are observing a hive in February or March, watch the incoming bees as they land before entering. You will see a little coloured swelling on each leg. These are the pollen-baskets, pockets on the legs which have been stuffed with pollen for passing on to the young bees. A seasoned bee-keeper quickly gets to know the sources of this pollen from its colours. The willow is a main source of early pollen in these latitudes.

While no complete analysis of pollen has yet been produced, enough is known of the effects of human consumption of pollen to say that, taken with honey, it is well-nigh the perfect food. Areas of the world where people live very long and active lives are characterised by a high consumption of honey from which the pollen has not been strained. Pollen has a protective function in the case of many diseases and a healing virtue in relation to others. Together with honey, propolis and royal jelly (these latter two also being products of the hive), pollen is effective against various bacteria, yeasts and fungi. Each of these will also curtail the multiplication of the flu virus. While it is popular to take honey in hot water for the onset of colds or influenza, it may be better simply to take it in its natural form; when heated it loses certain of its curative properties and the same is doubtless true of pollen. Natural, or beekeepers' honey, unstrained and containing pollen, wax, propolis and royal jelly in small amounts, is the ideal antidote to viral attacks of any kind. A course of pollen taken on its own in early winter is a defence against the various viral attacks to which you will be subject as the weather conditions deteriorate and the body defences are lowered.

As pollen is fairly strong stuff, it should be taken judiciously to begin with. A chemist with a feeling for natural cures will probably advise on frequency and amounts, but, as with honey, your own bodily requirements will soon inform you of how much to take.

Asthma, hay fever and allergies in general seem to go together, and they are all greatly helped by the taking of pollen internally. If you suffer from any of these, ask a beekeeper to save you the top skimmings of the honey before it is filtered for sale. The pollen grains and other medicinally useful substances will have floated to the top. A very little of this wonderful compendium of natural cures, if taken consistently for five or six weeks, will have results beyond your wildest expectations. You can purchase pollen tablets which will achieve much the same results, but it is always very hard to beat the completely natural product straight from the hive. Nobody knows why pollen taken in these forms has a healing effect on complaints often caused by pollen in the air in the first place, but many are sure from experience that it does work. Research is in progress to match various blends of the pollens of different flowers to the various related shades and grades of hay fever, allergies and asthmatic symptoms caused by these pollens.

Sufferers from rheumatism and arthritis have been known to gain relief from pollen taken over a period of three months or more. Some who improved significantly continued to take the pollen and have not had a return of the condition. Assuming these diseases to be the result of imbalances in the system, the main medicinal property of pollen seems to be its capacity to restore balance in the chemical constitution of the body.

But pollen — taken on its own or, preferably, in honey — has a particular contribution to make towards the treatment of an illness which is almost specific to our post-scientific world, namely radiation. Caused in the past by over-exposure to the sun's rays, in our time it has man-made sources, such as atomic bombs and the fall-out from atomic power stations. Loss of weight and of potency, nausea and vomiting, chronic tiredness, cancer and a frightening array of other life-threatening debilities are the results, and there is evidence to show that these have been reduced and in some cases have disappeared when fermented pollen and royal jelly were taken. It was remarked in Western Europe that for three perfectly good flying days bees had stayed firmly in their hives and could not be tempted out, when the Chernobyl nuclear accident was announced as having taken place three days previously. Such acute sensitivity to radiation must have some bearing on pollen's ability to combat the effects of radiation, though it is not yet understood. The results of further study of this extraordinary potential are anxiously awaited. A great many sufferers from radiation in Eastern Europe stand to benefit from taking pollen even while that work proceeds.

Pollen has a remarkable capacity to restore vitality and zest for living to people who have lost these essential accompaniments to health either through stress and strain or simply through the attrition of advancing years. Comfort-eating and drinking of refined food products can have a debilitating effect on all who indulge in it over a long — and sometimes not so long — period. The cream bun, the extra spoon of sugar in the coffee, the nip of whiskey or brandy to cheer us up: all of these, which seem so innocent on their own, add up to creeping bad dietary habits which must eventually take their toll. There is much misdirected discussion today on 'how much' of anything one can safely have. Often, the wrong question is being asked: it should be 'whether or not' rather than 'how much'. But help is at hand. Like its accompanying honey, pollen has marvellous restorative effects on the run-down or abused system. It pours all the right nutrients, vitamins, amino acids and minerals straight into your bloodstream and is good to take at all ages and stages of your life, while being especially appropriate for children and the elderly. Like honey, pollen is a first-class emergency food for anyone suffering from malnutrition or inability to ingest or hold food in any quantity.

If you follow athletics, you might be interested to learn that pollen plays an important part in the diet of probably a majority of Olympic athletes. As dietary effects are spread over comparatively long periods of time, athletes tend to take pollen constantly as a supplement so that they can be at peak fitness when the moment comes to compete. Professional athletes are keen students of the conditions most conducive to physical fitness, and are well aware of pollen's role in bringing muscles to the high tone required for competitive sport.

There is some trial and error involved in arriving at the type and dosage of pollen most appropriate to your condition or general state of health, but most of the pollens commercially available should be of benefit in many ways. The producers of pollen products may supply you with an amount of general information, and a medical herbalist will certainly be of help. It is not possible to be more specific in a book like this, but the remedial powers of pollen, and of all bee products, is a subject worthy of pursuit.

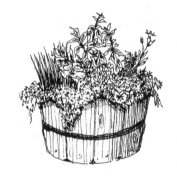

APPLE CIDER VINEGAR

Apple cider vinegar comes from the juice of apples. It is a great restorer and maintainer of health, containing as it does so many ingredients which the body needs — ingredients which are all too often refined out of food in manufacturing processes. One such is potassium, essential for growth and the renewal of tissues in the human body. Other important constituents include sodium, phosphorous, iron, sulphur and silicon. Cider vinegar combines extremely well with honey. Two teaspoonfuls of each, stirred well in a glass of water, taken with meals three times a day is as near as man will ever get to an elixir of life; and if honey on its own is too sweet for your taste, the cider vinegar will sharpen it for you. So popular is this mixture that you can buy it already made up in health food shops under the name of 'Honegar'. Be sure you get a brand which has real honey and not any of the substitutes, which are worse than useless.

Cider vinegar works by helping to keep in order your acid/alkaline balance, upon which the proper functioning of your body chemistry depends. In the process it strengthens the body's defences against disease. Taken internally, with or without honey, it is such a remarkable agent for good health that listed here are only some of its more significant benefits.

In cases of haemorrhaging, cider vinegar will renew the blood's ability to coagulate. Eczema is successfully treated by taking the honegar at meals while also applying well-diluted cider vinegar externally to the affected areas as many times each day as the patient wishes. Eczema sufferers often lack potassium, which the cider vinegar supplies. Salt irritates eczema and should be reduced in the daily diet. Cider vinegar is helpful in cases of high blood pressure as it thins the blood without impairing its ability to clot. If honey is taken at the same time, it reinforces the effect of the cider vinegar and, through its sedative virtues, also calms the nervous system, thereby countering one of the main causes of high blood pressure.

Hydrochloric acid both helps us to digest food and combats germs in the stomach. In our time, for a variety of reasons which includes the excessive strains of everyday life, the body's production of this important acid tends to be inadequate. This in its turn is sometimes erroneously diagnosed as hyperacidity — a shortage of acid unfortunately has exactly the same symptoms as a surplus — and wrongly treated with alkaline doses of one kind or another. The three-times-daily dose of honegar described above is usually the best response to feeling 'acidy'. Reduce the intake of protein until the acidic feeling disappears. Stomach ulcers may be associated with an excess of hydrochloric acid; honegar is not the answer to this problem but rather the reduction of protein food and an increased intake of fruit and salad vegetables. Try always to eat raw fruit rather than fruit from a can, which is generally afloat in the kinds of sugar that your system could cheerfully do without.

A tablespoonful of honey taken internally and the inhaled vapour of cider vinegar which has been boiled with an equal amount of water and allowed to cool, is often sufficient medication for a migraine headache. Insomnia is sometimes defeated if you take a glass of honegar before going to bed. Tartar formation on teeth can be reversed by constant recourse to cider vinegar, which will also reduce the risk of gum disease.

Arthritis is frequently caused by the uneven deposition of calcium on the joints, resulting in pain and discomfort. This happens because the calcium should have been kept in solution but was not in the acid medium required for this state. Cider vinegar supplies the necessary acid, acting in much the same way here as in the dissolution of tartar. Arthritic hands and feet can be bathed in a warmed solution of one part of cider vinegar to five parts of water; apply this solution to painful knee joints in a wet bandage held in place by a dry one. The process can be repeated as many times as required.

Superfluous fat is burnt off the body if one persistently takes the honegar solution; however, an unamended diet may continue to pile on the fat and make it next to impossible for the honegar to show results. The potassium in the honegar attracts surplus moisture and compels the body to expel this through sweating and urination. Provided that good diet is maintained, there will be a gradual but measurable reduction until proper weight is achieved. It is advisable to add a dash of daily exercise to the mix and to avoid any kind of so-called 'crash' dieting, which usually proves disastrous. Crash diets are not natural and, therefore, can only very briefly appear to be successful.

Disease-making bacteria in the intestines are best controlled by the daily dose of honegar. These bacteria can cause diarrhoea, colitis and other diseases if they gain the upper hand but are kept securely in check by honey and cider vinegar. Honey taken on its own backed up by a good 'shot' of honegar three times every day for the duration of the hay fever season, is a folk medicine antidote to hay fever by which many people swear.

Sore throats can often be remedied by gargling with cider vinegar, a teaspoonful to a glass of water. Be sure to swallow the mixture and catch the lurking infection lower down.

Cider vinegar has many benefits to confer on the skin when applied externally. The normal condition of the skin is acidic and the use of soap sometimes diminishes the natural acid and causes irritation. Diluted cider vinegar usually restores the skin to its proper condition and thereby removes the irritation.

Ringworm can be cured by applications of cider vinegar accompanied by the taking internally of doses of honegar. Administer the cider vinegar frequently to the affected places. Varicose veins will shrink over a period of several weeks if cider vinegar is applied and honegar taken internally.

Much more could be written on the virtues of cider vinegar. You are referred in particular to the work of Dr D.C. Jarvis, who studied the highly effective folk medicine of Vermont in the US and concluded that a daily intake of cider vinegar with honey is the single greatest aid to continuing good health that man has so far discovered or devised.

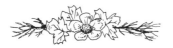

KELP

Kelp or bladderwrack, commonly and simply called seaweed, is a powerful source of healing. It grows freely on the rocks beneath the sea around our coasts and is flung in bundles on the beaches when the weather is rough and stormy. It is still gathered from the shore and used as a natural fertiliser, especially along the west coast of Ireland but also in places like the Channel Islands. There are fields where potatoes have been grown every year for upwards of a hundred years without rotation, purely because of the health brought to the soil by kelp. The crops grown in kelp are full of uncontaminated nutrition and it seems a pity that it is not applied throughout our market gardens to bring the health and wealth of the sea to our tables. No doubt the all-persuasive arguments of 'Economics' could be marshalled against this suggestion, but there's no arguing against the flavour of a potato grown in seaweed.

Fortunately the medicinal values of kelp have long been appreciated, whether imbibed directly by eating the weed itself, indirectly through fertilised vegetable crops, or, at a third remove, taken in powder or tablet form (available from chemists' or health food shops). Acknowledged by both orthodox and herbal medical systems for centuries, its homeopathic capacities are beginning to be better understood in our own time and, like honey and pollen, kelp continues to yield riches that were not even dreamt of by modern researchers exploring its mysteries. Also, like honey and pollen, kelp contains many of the vitamins and minerals essential to human health in the organic condition most suitable to absorption by our bodies. It is perhaps best known for its iodine content but it incorporates many more health-giving substances, including a very valuable sugar called fucose. This has been found to help reduce weight in some people who suffer from obesity, through its normalising influence on the thyroid gland. It will not remove weight from people who are already at or below their proper healthy bodyweight. In general terms, kelp is probably nature's best weight controller. Fucose exercises the same kind of normalising effect on many other organs and can be administered homeopathically for such abnormalities.

Kelp has a remedial effect on the pancreas. The problem of indigestion is sometimes caused by a sluggish pancreas, and kelp is known to clear up this particular complaint very quickly. In association with a proper diet, it is a remedy for nervous complaints of various kinds. Here, as so often, we are in the indeterminate area where mind acts on body and body reacts on mind. The 'normalising' effects of kelp on different organs reflect through the nervous system to the mind and bring a stability and ease which will in its turn be transmitted back to the organs, reinforcing the effects of the kelp. Irritability and general nervous tension place stress on the entire system and not least upon the heart, so kelp can also be viewed as a valuable heart medicine.

Pains in the neck and headaches can have strange and sometimes remote origins. Kelp is worth trying as a simple, safe cure for such miseries as it has worked wonders in some cases. Even migraine has been relieved by taking kelp. Disease of the colon or lower intestine can cause havoc in both body and brain and the problem is often treated with enemas and, misguidedly, with purgatives. There was a time when the malfunctioning colon was actually removed altogether to prevent it from spreading poisons through the bloodstream. Kelp is a marvellous stimulant of the colon, especially when mixed with blackstrap molasses. This combination of perfectly natural foods is emerging as a real antidote to autotoxaemia or self-poisoning resulting from the accumulation of poisons in the colon. Headaches may well be caused by this condition and may, therefore, be relieved by the mixture.

Kelp has a particularly beneficial effect on the liver by giving it the salts required for proper, efficient functioning and by cleansing it of toxins. It also clears obstructions in the gall bladder. The kidneys benefit from a regular intake of kelp, as does the prostate gland, source of so much suffering to older men. Kelp has even been known to normalise the prostate gland in men of advancing years who have never before taken it.

The connection between iodine deficiency and thyroid problems has been understood since the middle of the last century, and as kelp is a major source of 'natural' iodine, it is frequently taken for goitre or abnormal enlargement of that gland. The range of problems which can arise from abnormalities of the thyroid includes obesity, dry skin and hair, kidney disorders and slow growth in children.

Radish tops, celery, parsley and carrots, kelp and molasses are very beneficial for people who suffer from rheumatism. Proper elimination of food wastes, especially of acids, is the beginning of the curing process. Massive over-dosing with sodium compounds to counteract acidity is actually counterproductive. The cure is worse than the disease. An extremely useful natural laxative includes kelp, molasses and perhaps a little all-bran, taken in a glass of water. Linseed is also useful, a dessertspoonful at a time with a glass of water. For rheumatism the kelp should be taken with every meal.

The influence of kelp on the bloodstream is salutary, the iodine and mineral salt acting as a stabilising and balancing element. Kelp is nature's means of bringing us the health-giving riches of the sea. Taken sensibly, it will have a most invigorating effect on your entire body.

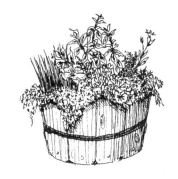

PART I

Herbs

AGRIMONY —
Agrimonia eupatoria
Part used: Herb

This tall spike, with myriad small, rose-shaped yellow flowerets (it is related to the rose) and large-toothed leaves, can be found growing in sunny waste places. Its height, usually 30 to 60 cm (1 to 2 feet) but sometimes 1.8 metres (6 feet) or more, has earned it the nickname of 'Church Steeples'. It is a perennial herb.

The whole plant yields a yellow dye which is darker the later in the year the plant is gathered, and which can be used to dye sheepswool. It is eaten by goats and sheep but avoided by other animals. The second part of the plant's scientific name commemorates King Mithridates Eupator of Pontus (136–63 BC), who is reported to have discovered its medicinal uses in classical times, so it could be said that its 'field trials' have continued now for a few thousand years.

Since the time of Mithridates, agrimony has been used, widely and with great success, to cure a variety of ailments. The Anglo Saxons applied it to heal warts, wounds and snake bites. In medieval France it was an ingredient in 'arquebusade water', which was administered to wounds inflicted by the arquebus or early hand-gun; it is still used in that country for bruises and sprains.

The herb's more general applications today include the alleviation of tonsillitis, thrush (or inflammation of the mucous membrane) in the mouth, anaemia, hardening of the liver, disorders of the spleen, lumbago and rheumatism. It is also effective against jaundice and is made into an ointment for varicose veins and ulcers of the lower leg.

Tonsillitis and other disorders of the mouth and throat are treated with a gargle of agrimony tea, which is made of the dried herb, leaves, flowers and stems. Swallow after gargling so that the liquid can reach the deepest infected areas and help prevent reinfection of the throat from below. Do not use agrimony internally while constipated.

ANGELICA—
Angelica archangelica
Parts used: Roots, leaves, seeds

Well known in early pagan times for its curative properties, this herb became associated with the feast of the Annunciation in Christian times, hence its name. Legend has it that angelica was revealed in a dream by an angel as the cure for a plague then raging. It is also said that it blooms on the feast-day of Michael the Archangel and it is therefore regarded as a sacred herb that wards off evil spirits. It is a perennial but goes through a three-year life cycle, flowering in the third year before it dies. However, severe cutting prolongs the life of this herb indefinitely.

The angelica can grow to 1.8 metres (6 feet) and has a very large root, which shares its magnificent aroma. Damp soil conditions suit this herb, though it is capable of finding its way in almost any environment.

The stem is frequently candied and used as green decoration on cakes and other confectionery. The stems when chewed give instant relief from flatulence. An infusion of the root also remedies flatulence and is a tonic for the bronchial tubes. Drying the yellow juice from the root and stem provides an effective medicine for rheumatism and gout. Indigestion, general debility and sluggishness are banished by the infused herb, two tablespoonfuls taken three or four times a day. A preparation of the roots was given to victims of typhoid fever in ancient times (this may account for the legend of the angel revealing it as a cure for the plague). Too much exposure of the skin to the juice of angelica can cause a skin rash; handle with care. Warning: angelica should not be given to people with diabetes as it causes an increase of sugar in the urine.

Herb as food
Angelica has a clean sharp flavour. It can be made into a syrup to liven up ice cream and fruit salads. The leaves can be cooked with sour fruit to remove its tartness, particularly rhubarb. For rhubarb pie, when you have lined the pie plate with the pastry and sprinkled a flour/sugar mixture over the crust, build layers of rhubarb and tender stems of angelica mixed with slices of lemon, each layer to be sprinkled with the flour/sugar. Cover with pastry and bake in the usual manner.

Crystallised angelica stems
Boil second-year fresh angelica stems. Remove from the water, strip outer skin and boil again until green but not too mushy. Drain the stems, weigh them and add half their weight of honey, cover and allow to stand overnight. Next day boil up the stems and honey and simmer for twenty minutes. Drain and dry the stems on greaseproof paper in a cool oven. Cool and store in airtight glass jars. Use for cake decorations.

Angelica and mint spread
Shred a mixture of fresh young angelica leaves and an equal amount of fresh mint leaves. Cover toasted wholemeal bread with mayonnaise and spread the herbs thickly on top.

APPLE —
Malus communis
Parts used: Fruit, bark

Ever since Eve tempted Adam the apple has been considered a health-enhancing food without equal; whether in Greek, Celtic or almost any other mythology, the apple holds a place of honour. Avalon, the dream city to which King Arthur was taken after he died, was really Ubhallan, 'The Place of Apples', from the Celtic (Irish) *ubhall* for 'apple'. As with so many plants and fruits, we find that ancient instincts are borne out, for the apple is indeed a manifold source of substances which will not alone cure but prevent a large number of human ailments.

Apples are best eaten first thing in the morning or last at night. An old rhyme holds that 'To eat an apple going to bed/Will make the doctor beg his bread.'

For coughs, hoarseness, lung, stomach and kidney diseases boil sliced apple with liquorice for twenty minutes. Drink the resultant decoction. For gout and rheumatism take a decoction of crushed, powdered apple peel three or four times a day. For hypertension, fatigue, shortage of minerals in the system, take two teaspoonfuls of apple cider vinegar and honey with water daily.

The bark of the apple tree will perform the same service as quinine in bringing down a fever. A mixture of the leaves, buds and flowers is said to relieve inflammation of the kidneys and also eliminate kidney stones and cystitis.

Apples help to clear the nose and sinuses of catarrh. They purify the blood and stimulate the digestion. They are also very beneficial to sufferers from arteriosclerosis, piles, obesity and diseases of the skin. The raw middle of an apple, rubbed against the affected area, brings great relief from itchy skin.

Herb as food
Elderberry and apple pie
For a treat in autumn when fruits are at their best, slice 450 g (1 lb) of cooking apples and combine with 225 g (½ lb) of elderberries stripped from their stalks. Put into a deep pie dish that has been lined with pastry. Add four tablespoonfuls of honey and a quarter-teaspoonful of cinnamon or ginger. Cover the pie with pastry and bake in the oven until golden-brown. Make it a really healthy dish by serving it with thick yoghurt, preferably homemade. Be sure to get to your elderberry tree before the birds realise the fruit is ripe, as birds are expert elderberry-strippers and can leave a tree naked in a matter of hours.

ASH —
Fraxinus excelsior
Parts used: Leaves, bark

So great was the respect of the ancient Teutons for the ash that they believed a giant ash tree supported the canopy of the heavens. Their spears had handles of ash, as had the spears of Homer's heroes of ancient Greece. The hurley is always made from ash specially grown. It is the toughest and most elastic of all timbers in Europe and one of the warmest and quickest to burn, even when green.

The ash has many medicinal applications. The bark stripped from the limbs in early spring was administered as a febrifuge before the discovery of quinine. It is still used as a remedy for intermittent fevers; it can be taken in powder form, or as a decoction, a cupful three times a day before meals.

Ash leaves are more active dried than fresh. They should be gathered from May to July. Infuse or mildly decoct, adding a few leaves of mint for aroma, for rheumatism, gout, renal colic and gravel. One cupful should be taken every three hours; to prevent further attack take 1 litre (1¾ pints) a day for fifteen days every two months. A mild infusion of ash leaves every morning is said to be a recipe for longevity.

The seeds of the ash have strong diuretic properties and are most effective in cases of dropsy. Make a mild decoction using 1 litre (1¾ pints) of water boiled for two or three minutes and sip it occasionally in the round of the day. Alternatively take it in powder form, approximately 10 g (⅓ oz) a day, mixed with honey or stirred into a drink.

BALM (LEMON BALM) —
Melissa officinalis
Part used: Herb

The balm, a low-growing shrubby plant, is widely thought the sweetest-smelling herb of all. Its aroma accounts for the alternative name, 'Lemon Balm'. *Melissa* is the Greek word for 'bee' and is said to have been applied to the plant because of its alleged attraction for bees. However, I have had lemon balm and bees in the same garden for many years and have never seen a bee on the plant. Is this an ancient error that has been repeated through two millennia? Fortunately, the rest of the information on the plant, given below, is well attested.

Balm is known to be good for the brain, especially the memory. It is also helpful in dispelling gloom and melancholy. The juice of the balm closes green wounds. In common with that of several other plants, its oil makes first-class dressing for cuts, depriving germs of oxygen and forcing them to leave. It then dries and seals the wound against unwelcome foreign bodies. Taken as an infusion, balm induces a light perspiration and has a cooling effect on people with influenza or heavy colds. Balm tea is pleasant to the taste; though sometimes flavoured with honey, this seems unnecessary for all except the sweetest-toothed. The plant dies back in winter, but its root is perennial and will send up vigorous new shoots in the spring. The balm is worth growing for its scent alone.

Herb as food

The leaves of the lemon balm are sometimes used to sweeten dishes. They have a particularly agreeable effect when chopped finely and sprinkled on fruit salads. They combine well with other herbs, particularly if a light — rather than a bitter — lemon taste is required.

Make a cool drink for the dog days of summer by mixing equal quantities of apple juice and lemonade with the juice of half a lemon, half a dozen balm leaves and the same number of mint leaves crushed. Stir together in a jug and serve.

For a tasty jelly stir honey, lemon and balm leaves into 15 g (½ oz) of gelatine that is dissolving in 150 ml (¼ pint) of hot water. Add 450 ml (¾ pint) of milk as the mixture cools. Allow to set and serve.

For roast duck stuffing mix a handful of lemon balm leaves with peeled, chopped cooking apples and an equal quantity of stoned prunes. This stuffing is delicious and helps to tenderise the bird.

If possible always use lemon balm fresh. The leaves can be picked from the plant all summer long. If you wish to dry this herb for later consumption use only the first cut. It tastes good in egg dishes, especially omelettes, and goes well with vegetables of all kinds.

BASIL, SWEET —
Ocimum basilium
Part used: Herb

This tall plant with grey-green leaves is an annual herb. A native of India, where it is held in high regard, it has a disinfecting and invigorating effect on malarious or fetid air and consequently is revered as the protecting spirit of the family in the homes of the Hindu people. In the past all Hindu families made daily offerings of rice and flowers to the basil.

The value of basil for flavouring soups and sauces has been known in the West since very early times; it has undoubted digestive properties as well as a marvellous flavour and aroma. Its medical uses arise mainly from its sedative and anti-spasmodic properties. Basil can have beneficial results when taken, even in food, by anyone with a nervous predisposition, and is helpful in the alleviation of vertigo, migraines and, in

some instances, insomnia. An infusion of basil in boiling water stops vomiting and eases nausea. The seeds were once thought to cure serpent bites and are still used to remove warts. A few drops of the sap from the leaves is reputed to ease earache. The powdered dried leaves make a snuff which helps to clear the nasal passages and restore the sense of smell. In some parts of Africa basil is given to children to rid them of worms.

An infusion should be taken three times a day, after meals, for all the complaints listed above (except earache and blocked nasal passages).

Herb as food
Basil is somewhat reminiscent of cloves in flavour. The taste intensifies when it is cooked, as does the aroma. It can enliven dull vegetables, soups and eggs; rice and tomatoes also gain from its inclusion. Casseroles of veal, beef, venison, lamb and game will improve with a little basil, but use with care: one or two leaves are generally sufficient for any dish. Basil has fresh leaves throughout the summer. A piece will keep in the deep-freeze but it doesn't dry well.

The classic sauce for all pasta dishes comes from Genoa and is called pesto. Take four tablespoonfuls of fresh chopped basil leaves, two tablespoonfuls of ground walnuts, three garlic cloves (crushed), three table-spoonfuls of Parmesan cheese, five tablespoonfuls of olive oil and two tablespoonfuls of melted butter. Pound together the basil, nuts and garlic, then add to grated cheese and mix well together. Add butter and oil slowly, blending thoroughly. Serve warm or cold to taste.

For a sauce which goes extremely well with both ox-tongue and roast pork add 225 ml (8 fl oz) of tomato purée to a pan of 225 g (½ lb) of freshly fried mushrooms. Return the pan to the heat and put in one tablespoonful each of chopped parsley, chopped tarragon and freshly chopped basil. Heat through and serve.

The seeds of basil make cool drinks more refreshing. Chew them as you drink.

BEDSTRAW, LADY'S —
Galium verum
Parts used: Flowering tops

The more common name of this herb, 'Our Lady's Bedstraw', comes from the legend that it was in the hay of the manger at Bethlehem. However that may have been, it was certainly used by ladies of the manor from the Middle Ages on to stuff pillows and mattresses. Another of its local names, the 'Cheese Rennet', derives from its ability to curdle milk.

The herb is still in use medicinally, particularly as a cure for gravel and other diseases of the urinary tract. In the days when people walked a great deal or travelled long distances on horseback, the bedstraw was made into an ointment to rub on sore bones and joints. It once enjoyed a popular reputation as a cure for epilepsy. The juice, like that of so many other herbs, had both a stimulating and a healing effect when applied to the skin. A decoction of the bedstraw was sometimes given to stop a bleeding nose and to heal internal wounds. Stomach pains, hysteria and vertigo are remedied by the herb, and its diuretic properties are said to be of particular benefit in cases of obesity and in the treatment of various skin diseases.

The root of the bedstraw yields a red dye suitable for woollen materials, but as the crop per acre is very small the amounts are not commercial. Perhaps it will give that tired old garment of yours a top-of-the-market look — at least it will be exclusive.

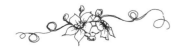

Herb as food

If you use the bedstraw to make cheese and find it less effective at curdling milk than you might wish, add a little of the juice of the stinging nettle, preferably picked before the beginning of June as it will be too acidic after that.

BILBERRY —
Vaccinium myrtillus
Parts used: Ripe fruit and leaves

Fraughan Sunday or the Sunday nearest to 1 August is the day on which, from time immemorial, entire families take to the mountains and the bogs to gather this, the first and the best fruit of the year. No plant has more names than this undershrub, which is found mainly wherever heather grows and whose fruit resembles the blackcurrant. There are still celebrations in many country places on Fraughan Sunday, or Garlic Sunday or even Garland Sunday as it is variously called; a carnival spirit prevails, courtships blossom and, no doubt in the hope of a good harvest, matches are made. The bilberries will remain ripe until the middle of September, even later on sunny, heathery, south-facing mountainsides. Let us hope the matches made on Garland Sunday endure longer again.

But the bilberry is not just a romantic throwback to the ancient world. On the contrary, it has at least one medicinal use which makes it essential to survival on our overcrowded roads: the skin of the berry contains a substance that improves night vision. Among their other remarkable qualities, the berries are strongly disinfectant and have been proven capable of sterilising the typhoid bacillus within twenty-four hours. They are nature's cure for acute enteritis, dysentery, diarrhoea and other bowel disorders.

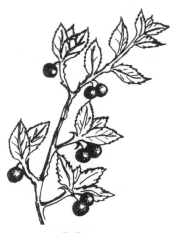

Bilberry

The berries are dried in the shade and will keep for a year. They can be chewed and swallowed (chew them for as long as you can), or decocted. The decoction has additional uses as a gargle for disorders of the throat and as a lotion for skin complaints. It can be helpful applied as a compress for haemorrhoids.

A decoction of the leaves is beneficial for cystitis, bed-wetting among children, eczema and pruritus. It lowers the blood sugar level — taken either on its own or in a decoction with an equal amount of strawberry leaves — and therefore makes a welcome contribution to the control of diabetes.

The juice of the berries produces an indelible dye of blue or purple which has been used for centuries on woollen cloth. The leaves of the bilberry have been both added to and substituted for Indian tea.

Herb as food

Bilberry fritter
In late summer or early autumn this makes an unusual dish. Generously grease an oven-proof dish with butter. Mix together in a bowl 300 ml (½ pint) of milk, 110 g (4 oz) of flour, one tablespoon of honey, the yolks of two eggs and 225 g (½ lb) of washed bilberries. Whisk the egg whites stiffly and fold into the bilberry batter. Pour into the buttered dish and bake in a hot oven until well risen and golden-brown. Serve immediately with some more honey poured over it.

Stewed bilberries
Add two tablespoonfuls of honey to 225 g (½ lb) of bilberries and two tablespoonfuls of water and cook gently in a covered pan for a delicious dessert or breakfast.

BIRCH —
Betula alba
Parts used: Bark, leaves

This most useful of trees is made into broom handles, staves for herring barrels, clogs, roofing for huts (in Lapland and Sweden), cord, baskets, nets, plates and an endless list of other items essential to those living in the more northerly regions of the world. Of all trees the birch grows furthest north, one reason being its flexibility in strong gales. When next you see Russian leather, note its lovely quality and the distinctive scent imparted to it by the oil of birch tar. Books bound in this leather are much less inclined to go mouldy.

The sap of the birch has long been considered, as Baron Percy, inspector general of the medical service of Napoleon's armies, declared, 'an invaluable cure for rheumatic diseases, bladder obstructions and numberless chronic sicknesses against which medical science is so prone to fail'. This sap should be taken from the birch in spring by boring a small hole in the bark of the trunk, inserting a straw and collecting it in a covered container. Don't forget to plug the hole afterwards. If you cannot find an available birch, all is not lost. A decoction of birch leaves, gathered in the spring and dried away from the sunlight, will be just as good for you. A pinch of bicarbonate of soda, added when the decoction has cooled a little, helps the beneficial elements in the leaves to dissolve. Let the mixture infuse for some hours before you take it. Four cupfuls of this tea, which is strongly diuretic, should be taken between meals each day to gain relief from skin diseases, fluid retention, rheumatism, gout, cardiac and renal oedema and stones in the kidney and bladder. Use this tea also as a cleansing compress for

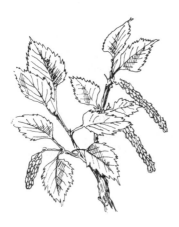

Birch

eczema, pimples, acne and other facial blemishes. To sleep in a warm bed full of dry birch leaves is said to relieve rheumatism, arthritis and various congestive conditions.

BLACKBERRY —
Rubus fructicosus
Parts used: Roots, leaves and berries

This hedgerow favourite is mentioned in the Bible as the king of trees and was known to the ancient Greeks as a cure for gout. The bramble cure for various ailments in times past consisted of the sufferer crawling or being dragged under a rooted blackberry offshoot, sometimes to the accompaniment of a spoken charm or spell. Hernia in small children and boils were said to benefit from such unorthodox treatment. Watch carefully where the birds pick their blackberries, and follow their example. You will find that the berries will be neither too sweet nor too tart, but just the right combination.

A decoction made from dried blackberry leaves is a remedy for inflammation of the mouth and of the mucous membranes of the digestive tract. Gastritis, dysentery, diarrhoea and enteritis are all relieved by taking four cupfuls each day between meals;

this is also useful for piles and cystitis. Sore throats are alleviated by gargling with blackberry decoction. Blackberry jam, so delicious and nourishing on our autumn and winter tables, is also medically beneficial for irritation of the vocal cords, hoarseness or indeed any affliction of the throat. Take a few tablespoonfuls the day of your Christmas party; you will find yourself in excellent voice when called upon to deliver your party piece.

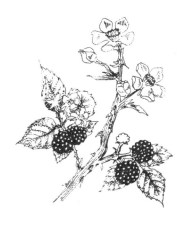

Blackberry

Herb as food

Blackberry ice cream

For a delicious dessert for late summer parties and celebrations take 900 g (2 lbs) of ripe blackberries, 600 ml (1 pint) of thick cream, the juice of a lemon and four tablespoonfuls of liquid honey. Crush the blackberries and press through a sieve to remove the seeds. Add the lemon juice and honey to the blackberry juice. Whip the cream and fold it into the blackberry mixture and freeze as for any homemade ice cream.

Blackberry bake

A hot dessert made with blackberries is a must for slightly colder days of early autumn. Make a topping by beating together 85 g (3 oz) of butter with four tablespoonfuls of honey. Add one egg, 110 g (4 oz) of wholemeal flour and two teaspoonfuls of baking powder, then mix in enough milk to make a soft batter. Put 450 g (1 lb) of blackberries into a deep greased pie dish with two tablespoonfuls of honey and the juice of a lemon. Pour the batter over the blackberries and bake in the oven until golden-brown.

Spiced blackberry jelly

This can accompany meat dishes, both hot and cold. To 900 g (2 lbs) of blackberries add the juice of a lemon, one teaspoon of ground ginger, half a teaspoon of ground cinnamon, three or four whole cloves and one cup of cider vinegar. Put them in a saucepan and heat slowly until the berries are soft. Press the berries from time to time so that the juice runs out freely. Drip through a jelly-bag overnight and measure the juice in the morning. To each 600 ml (1 pint) of juice add 450 g (1 lb) of sugar. Return to the saucepan and heat until the sugar has dissolved, then boil for about five minutes or until the jelly reaches setting point. Pour into heated jars and cover in the usual way.

Blackberry omelette

Separate two eggs, put the yolks into a bowl with one dessertspoonful of liquid honey and mix them well together. Beat the egg whites until stiff and fold into the egg yolk mixture. Melt a tablespoonful of butter in a clean pan and pour on the egg mixture to make an omelette. When the omelette is cooked spread half of it with a cupful of ripe blackberries lightly crushed until the juice is just running out of them. Fold over the omelette and serve. The slight tartness and unique flavour of the blackberries are a delightful complement to the omelette.

BLACKCURRANT —
Ribes nigrum
Parts used: Fruit, leaves, bark, roots

If there is a wet corner in your garden and you are wondering what to plant there, spare a thought for the blackcurrant. It is, after all, happiest when in the wild state, in marshy woodland, and of all shrubs it concentrates the most vitamin C. It relieves a very wide number of ailments, the leaves being quite as effective as the currants.

Arthritis, rheumatism, oedema, general fatigue and difficulties of the urinary tract are all improved by an infusion of the leaves, which is diuretic. This also makes a refreshing summer drink. For an anti-rheumatic remedy, infuse two parts of dry blackcurrant leaves to one part each of dried flowerheads of meadowsweet and dry ash leaves. Take one tablespoonful of this infusion in a cup of boiling water each night.

The juice of the blackcurrant fruit boiled to an extract with sugar (called rob) is a remedy for inflammation of the throat. Lozenges prepared from this extract are particularly beneficial for throat ailments and are available in chemists' shops.

Blackcurrant jelly made from the fruit has long been treasured for helping sufferers from colds. It should not contain too much sugar as this will reduce its medicinal potency. It acts as a laxative and also has a cooling effect. Blackcurrant tea is made by putting a tablespoonful of the jelly in a tumbler of boiling water. Drink it hot several times in the day and your cold and its accompanying misery will quickly pass. If you are bitten by insects while picking the fruit of the blackcurrant, just take a few leaves of the shrub, squeeze them together and rub the juice on the bites. You'll be surprised at the relief this provides — just as the dock leaves remedy the nettle sting.

BORAGE —
Borago officinalis
Parts used: Leaves, flowers

The beautiful blue star-shaped flower of the borage is familiar to all gardeners. It has long been one of man's best friends in the plant kingdom, for it has the special quality of raising one's spirits. The English herbalist John Gerard (1545–1612) wrote: 'The leaves and flowers of Borage put into wine make men and women glad and merry and drive away all sadness, dullness and melancholy.' The Greeks made a cure for alcoholic hangovers from it. According to Homer, borage steeped in wine brought complete forgetfulness. The plant yields nectar from which bees make magnificent honey.

Borage is very effective against fevers and against pulmonary ailments when cooked as a vegetable. The stem and leaves are more active than the flower; therefore the whole plant should be gathered. A decoction taken four or five times a day is good for all contagious fevers such as influenza, chicken-pox, scarlet fever and measles. The flowers, when candied, are supposed to help build up convalescing patients. The juice in syrup was anciently thought to be effective against jaundice, ringworm and itch. The dried herb was never used then, only the green. 'And yet', Nicholas Culpeper (1616–54) wrote, 'the ashes thereof boiled in mead or honeyed water, is available in inflammation and ulcers of the mouth and throat, as a gargle.' Borage is an ingredient of Pimms Number One.

Herb as food
The flavour of borage is somewhat like that of cucumber. Its leaves and flowers in sprays are favourite garnishings for claret cups and punch. The flowers can be crystallised and the tender leaves go well with cottage cheese, fish salads and new potatoes.

Borage flower syrup
Take this tasty light syrup when you are tired (perhaps a tablespoonful) or add it to fruit salads. Cover the flowers with boiling water, put a cloth over the container and leave to steep overnight. Go to the garden for

fresh flowers the next day. Strain and boil the liquid from the previous day's flowers and pour it over the fresh-picked flowers. Cover and allow to steep for ten hours. Press, strain and measure the resulting liquid. Stir in 450 g (1 lb) of sugar to every 600 ml (1 pint) of liquid over a low heat and when the sugar has melted boil for five minutes. Skim and leave to cool. Bottle cold, cork tightly and store in a cool place.

BUGLE, COMMON —
Ajuga reptans
Part used: Herb

The common bugle is found in damp meadows and among woods. It grows flower-stalks from 15 to 23 cm (6 to 9 inches) tall and has long creeping runners with pairs of leaves here and there. The flowers are blue to light purple and the whole plant presents a very handsome appearance.

In olden days the bugle was highly esteemed for its powers of healing, and it is still considered to have some medicinal virtue. Known to arrest haemorrhages, it is given as an infusion to people who are coughing blood in incipient consumption. It is a very good and a very agreeable remedy for those who have drunk to excess. A decoction of the common bugle is a cure for quinsy. A decoction of the leaves and flowers in wine is thought to dissolve the blood congealed in people who have fallen or otherwise been internally injured. A poultice of bruised leaves reputedly cures sores and ulcers and gangrene; for better effect add honey. Like the comfrey the bugle, either taken internally or applied externally, helps broken bones to knit. An ointment made with common bugle leaves and scabious and sanicle is a defence against bruises, cuts and other accidental damage that every household would be advised to keep in store. An infusion of the leaves acts as a mild laxative. Bugle is closely related to the wood sanicle.

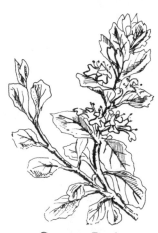

Common Bugle

BURDOCK —
Arctium lappa
Parts used: Root, herb and seeds (fruits)

Burdock is that large plant which gives children sticky fruits to hang on each other's clothes. The little hooks by which it clings to clothing fulfil the function, when stuck on the coats of animals, of carrying the burdock across long distances to where it can commence new colonies.

The dried roots, the fruits and leaves are all used medicinally. The burdock, like the nettle, is a great purifier of the blood. It is good for all skin conditions and is known to have cured eczema; the root taken as a decoction is the standard remedy in these situations. For boils, ulcers and various other skin disorders the decoction of the root can be taken both internally and externally. An infusion of the leaves is a good conditioner for a weak stomach, and a poultice of the leaves boiled briefly in slightly salty water is of benefit for bruises. A decoction of the root lowers the blood sugar level and therefore assists diabetics. An infusion of the root taken with almost an equal part of milk and sweetened with a little honey is a remedy for rheumatism, arthritis and gout. Apply poultices of the fresh leaves at the same time as taking this infusion, morning and evening. King Henry III is said to have been cured of an unmentionable disease by the burdock. An infusion of the seeds is held by many to be a good cure for kidney stone.

If the plant is cut before the flower opens it makes a delicious vegetable similar in taste to the asparagus and also a most acceptable salad. It is gently laxative.

CAMOMILE —
Anthemis nobilis
Parts used: Flowers, herb

The ancient Egyptians dedicated the camomile to their sun god, so highly did they value its medicinal properties. The Greeks gave it the name, which means 'ground-apple', because it smells just like a ripe, sweet apple. The Spaniards flavour one of their lightest sherries with it and call it 'manzarilla', 'little apple'. It is a low-growing, trailing plant whose flower is golden-yellow centred with white petals rather like a large daisy. The ripe apple aroma masks a taste which some find bitter. There are both wild and cultivated varieties.

The whole plant is medically valuable, but the flower is the part of highest quality and the most generally used. There are single (wild) and double (cultivated) flowers, each of which contains a strong alkali which could destroy the coating of stomach and bowels if drunk to excess. The double flowers contain far less, however, and so they alone are used.

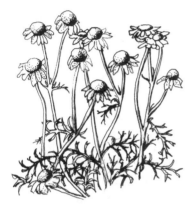

Camomile

Notwithstanding this cautionary note, an infusion of the cultivated camomile flower is an excellent treatment for hysteria and other nervous manifestations. Reassuring and sedative, it will prevent a full attack of delirium tremens if taken at an early stage, enjoys a high reputation as a remedy for nightmares, and can relieve the symptoms of pre-menstrual tension. Always prepare the infusion in a covered vessel or much of the medicinal potency will be lost in evaporation. For old

people the infusion, or camomile tea as it is called, taken cold, has a very appetising effect. It is also beneficial in cases of colic, indigestion, heartburn and general sluggishness of the system. Camomile has been used for thousands of years by blonde women as a hairwash. It is the original provider of 'highlights'.

CATMINT —
Nepeta cataria
Parts used: Leaves, herb

The catmint has an aroma somewhat like that of the pennyroyal and the mint which, for some reason, renders it magnetically attractive to cats. If the herb is bruised, releasing more of its aroma than usual, cats will destroy it in their anxiety to be close to it. Rats, on the other hand, dislike it intensely and it has therefore been grown as a protecting screen around other, more valuable crops. Catmint makes a handsome plant for a border or rock garden.

Catmint tea has the power to draw perspiration freely from a person with a fever; it also brings on sleep and is beneficial in relation to nervousness of any kind. It should always be infused as boiling does not suit its rather volatile characteristics. Catmint will reduce swellings if it is applied either as a fomentation or as a poultice. It can relieve coughing, especially if sweetened by a little honey. The green leaves bruised and made into an ointment make a remedy for piles. Catmint has a particular value as a treatment for nervous headache. It is preferable in this case not to take it as a tea but to express (or squeeze) the juice out of the green herb and take a tablespoonful three times each day. The young tops of catmint made into a conserve have been known to remedy nightmares. If planting catmint, you are advised to raise it from seed. For some strange reason cats almost invariably destroy the transplanted herb but never trouble one that comes up from seed.

COLTSFOOT —
Tussilago farfara
Parts used: Leaves, flowers, roots

The coltsfoot has long stalks, hoof-shaped leaves and a yellow flower. It should not be confused with the butterbur, which it resembles. The parts used for medicinal purposes are the leaves gathered in June and, sometimes, the flower-stalks gathered in February. It is a very difficult plant to control in gardens or pastures owing to its habit of suddenly springing up after ground has been disturbed.

The coltsfoot is one of the most commonly sought-after remedies for coughing. It is usually combined, for this purpose, with other herbs with pectoral characteristics, e.g. horehound or ground ivy. British herb tobacco, which is thought to benefit a bad chest, has coltsfoot as its main ingredient. Those who labour under asthmatic or bronchial conditions and other lung problems report much relief from smoking this. But, while it is believed to have no ill effects, it is a brave doctor who would now recommend any kind of smoking. A decoction of coltsfoot, possibly sweetened with a little honey, relieves both asthma and colds. Coltsfoot tea will have the same effect and coltsfoot rock, when it can be obtained, is a sound, safe cure for coughs. Syrup of coltsfoot is a known remedy for chronic bronchitis, wheezing and shortness of breath.

Distilled water of coltsfoot and elderflowers is effective in cases of fever when accompanied by the application to the head of cloths dipped in the distillation. These cloth compresses are also useful for inflammations or hot 'angry' swellings and for erysipelas. Warning: the appearance of this plant varies at different stages of its life cycle. Exercise extreme caution when identifying it.

COMFREY —
Symphytum officinale
Parts used: Roots, leaves

This tall-growing plant with drooping one-sided clusters of off-white or purple flowers and large hairy leaves is related to the borage. One of the most important of the herbs for many reasons, it likes to grow in damp places but is found very generally in various locations and conditions. Comfrey is grown on a field scale as a forage crop for animals and also as a vegetable for human consumption. In the latter capacity it is particularly popular in Japan.

It is still possible to find comfrey growing beside old and ruined cottages in remote places because in the days when medical services were sparse and difficult of access it was used, both applied as an external poultice and taken internally, to heal fractured bones — hence its popular name 'Knitbone'. The leaves of the comfrey are marvellously effective as an external remedy, both as a poultice for deep cuts and to draw boils and abscesses, and as a fomentation for administration to bruises, swellings and sprains. Applied to a fracture, the leaves reduce the surrounding swelling, thereby facilitating the joining up of the fractured parts.

Comfrey is very beneficial to sufferers from lung troubles and whooping cough. It is highly regarded for consumption and bleeding of the lung. A decoction of the comfrey leaf is of great value to sufferers from asthma and hay fever and can be taken in small amounts at the patient's discretion. The same rule applies here as in all cases of herbal preparations: it is not the volume of the remedy that matters so much as its suitability to the repair of the particular ailment.

Herb as food
Comfrey soup
This is nourishing (the leaves are full of vitamins and minerals) and has a strong vegetable taste. Take two cupfuls of young comfrey leaves, soak them for a few minutes in cold water, then wash them and discard any tough bits. Slice an onion and cook in a little butter or oil in a saucepan until it is soft, then shake a dessertspoonful of flour over the onion in the pan. Stir in the flour and gradually add 600 ml (1 pint) of

stock; keep stirring until the soup thickens. Add the comfrey leaves and simmer for about half an hour, then put the soup through a liquidiser.

Comfrey as vegetable
Pick young fresh leaves and, when cooked, liquidise and add a generous dollop of thick cream. Serve hot. This mixture can be very good when cooked in savoury flans.

CORNFLOWER—
Centaurea cyanus
Part used: Flowers

The cornflower is one of the loveliest of the herbs encountered in the wild. It is called after the centaur Chiron, who was credited in Greek mythology with having taught to mankind the art of herbal healing. The extremely tough stem gave the flower its least complimentary nickname, 'Hurt Sickle', for its habit of taking the edges off sickles. The flowers are of a distinctive bright blue colour and are the part used in herbal preparations.

A decoction of the cornflower is recommended for treatment of sore eyes. Conjunctivitis and general irritation of the eye are said to be improved or remedied by the application of cold compresses of the decoction or by using it as an eyewash. There is a semi-legendary notion that the cornflower is more effective in treating blue eyes, presumably because of its colour, and that likewise the plantain is better for dark eyes. Unlikely as this prescription may seem, stranger things are known to be true in the herb world. At any rate let it be recorded that a well-known and widely respected eyewash called 'Eau de Casselunettes' was once made from the petals of the cornflower.

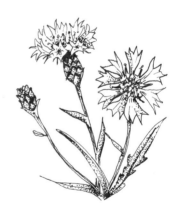

Cornflower

A decoction of the cornflower is also known to make a beauty treatment that gives firmness and tone to the skin. It is believed to have its virtues for treatment of various problems in the mouth, e.g. gingivitis. An infusion of the dried flowers may be taken internally for rheumatism and gout and for kidney problems. Its seeds have been used as a remedy for jaundice. They are purgative and so should be treated with caution.

Couch Grass —
Agropyrum repens
Part used: Rhizome (underground stem)

Many of us will have heard couch or scutch grass being spoken about in the most uncomplimentary terms by both farmers and gardeners. Under whatever name, switch, scutch or couch, it is the least popular — because it is the most invasive — of all the unwanted visitors to tilled soil. Its underground stem creeps quickly along, just below the surface of loosened earth, ramifying into an endless succession of branches, spreading in all directions at once and eating up a great deal of the natural nutrition that should be going into the farmer's field crop or the vegetables in the gardener's patch. Only the constant trampling of animals at pasture can make the soil firm enough to stop the onward march of the couch.

And yet, for all its plunder of the soil's nourishment — or perhaps because of it — the couch has many useful medicinal qualities which make it a herb of high standing among those who appreciate its true worth and function. It has even been ground to a flour to make bread during shortages of wheat flour in the past.

Couch is called the dog-grass because dogs seek it out when they are sick. The juice of the roots is good for the liver and alleviates jaundice. A decoction of the roots has a purifying effect on the blood if taken in early spring. Cystitis and diseases of the bladder are greatly relieved by this decoction; so are cases of gravel and other irritations of the urinary passage. Take wineglassful doses of the decoction cold in cases of rheumatism and gout. In preparation, remove all traces of rootlets from the rhizome, as well as all leaves. The cleaned rhizome or underground stem alone is used in medicine. You won't have any difficulty in finding whatever quantity you desire, once you've learnt to recognise it. Ask any farmer or gardener; they may even pay you to remove it.

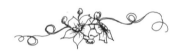

COWSLIP —
Primula veris
Part used: Yellow corolla
(plucked from green calyx)

The cowslip needs no introduction, even to the most infrequent visitor to the countryside. Many will know that it was anciently thought to hold a secret recipe to beautify the complexion. It has religious associations too, being known at one time as Herb Peter and the Key Flower owing to the similarity between its pendent flowers and a bunch of keys, the traditional emblem of St Peter. Cowslips were once eaten in salads and a delicious wine is made from their flowers.

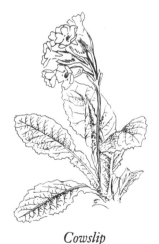

Cowslip

But the herb has more serious medical uses, despite the fact that only the yellow corolla is used, no green part being considered necessary. An infusion made with loaf sugar to a thin yellow syrup is supposed to assist in cases of nervous debility brought on by excitement. It was formerly thought to be helpful in paralytic ailments and was also held to be beneficial to a failing memory. The secret of the remedy for blemishes of the complexion was simply to bathe the face with the expressed juice of the flower. Sometimes the flowers were sprinkled with white wine before the juice was extracted. Decoction of cowslip has a soothing, soporific effect taken before going to bed. If you are picking cowslips for purposes of making up any of the remedies described above, be sure to leave the main plant in the ground, removing only the part required. Also — and this applies especially to all herbs picked for internal use — be sure they come from a place which has not been sprayed with insecticide or herbicide or drowned in artificial fertiliser. Residents of the poorer counties have the advantage here, as their farmers can't afford to poison their environment. Pick the herbs as far away as possible from roads and from sources of industrial pollution. Although nowhere is safe nowadays, some places are safer than others.

DAISY, COMMON —
Bellis perennis
Parts used: Root, leaves

Even the daisy — the least, yet in some ways the loveliest of common plants — is a friend to man. Why do people make such efforts to banish it from their gardens? It spreads and spreads, they say, until there is no grass left. So, what's wrong with a lawnful of daisies? Maybe familiarity has bred contempt. If the daisy were a rare exotic flower to be found only on high mountain ledges or in perilous bogs, we would search it out diligently and treasure it. Before we are so foolish as to dismiss the common daisy, let us look at the virtues which made it a friend to our ancestors before modern medicine arrived with its 'pill for every ill'.

A distilled water from the daisy taken internally was a remedy for inflammations of the liver. An infusion of the leaves was used to bring down fevers. The daisy was one ingredient in an ointment for gouts, fevers and wounds which was popular 500 years ago and more. A strong decoction of the roots was taken as a cure for scurvy. In Scotland the daisy was known as the 'Bairnwort' or children's flower for the plea-sure children took in making daisy chains. So like the sun in miniature is it that, on the authority of Geoffrey Chaucer, we believe it is named the 'day's eye'.

Well by reason men it call maie
The Daisie or else the Eye of the
Daie.

DAISY, OX-EYE —
Chrysanthemum leucanthemum
Parts used: Whole herb, flowers, root

This tall-growing flower of fairly general occurrence is to be seen from about late May until the end of June and sometimes later. At first sight it looks like a large daisy. The people of ancient times considered it very useful in women's complaints. In Christian times it was variously dedicated to St Mary Magdalene and St John. The ox-eye daisy is one of the chrysanthemum family.

The whole herb is used medicinally and also the flowers separately. Asthma and whooping cough have been successfully treated with the ox-eye daisy, as have night sweats. The flowers, given in infusion, have a relieving effect on coughs and catarrh. The root is also sometimes used for night sweats in pulmonary consumption. Jaundice is said to be relieved by an infusion of the flowers. Either an infusion or a decoction can be applied to bruises and wounds. Ointments and syrups can be made with the herb, the ointment being particularly effective — when it is made of a combination of agrimony and ox-eye daisy – for reducing inflammation around wounds, cuts and lacerations of the skin. The bruised leaves will achieve much the same result but cannot be stored for future use. The young leaves of the ox-eye daisy are sometimes eaten in Mediterranean lands, but, as they are very bitter to the taste, it would be difficult to recommend them here where, unlike the peoples of southern Europe, we are not trained since childhood to grazing on such health-giving herbs.

DANDELION —
Taraxacum officinale
Parts used: Root, leaves

The familiar yellow flower of the dandelion is found far and wide from spring right through to autumn. During this time it gives forth a continuous flow of pollen and nectar, filling all the gaps between the flowering times of less generous flowers and shrubs. No wonder it is considered the beekeeper's most prolific and most loyal friend.

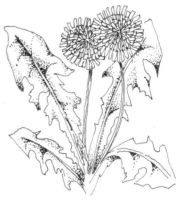

Dandelion

The uses of the dandelion are endless. The leaves can be eaten as salad or boiled as a vegetable. Dandelion coffee made from the roots of the herb has grown in popularity in recent years and is readily available in health food shops. A mixture of a little real coffee can produce a very interesting taste. To make your own dandelion coffee, dig the roots in good soil in the autumn and take those roots which are least divided. Wash them thoroughly, dry in artificial heat, roast and then grind them. Do not cut them as you will lose the valuable milky juice which contains their medicinal elements. Dandelion coffee provides us with a far healthier drink than that which we usually call coffee. It does not contain caffeine and although it is diuretic it has the great virtue of replacing the potassium which is usually lost through the action of other diuretic drinks.

Because the leaves of the dandelion are rich in iron and good for anaemia, they help clear up imperfections of the skin and are effective in dissolving the chalky deposits left on the bone joints by rheumatoid arthritis. Tea made from either fresh or dried dandelion leaves is good for all digestive upsets.

The heart, the stomach, the bladder, the kidneys and the liver all derive healthy stimulation from the dandelion. It makes a welcome and refreshing addition to any diet and could be just the thing to give new delight to a jaded palate. How foolish are those who call this most useful of herbs a weed!

Herb as food
Dandelion soup
Take a basin full of dandelion leaves, 30 g (1 oz) of butter, one onion, one potato and 1.1 litres (2 pints) of stock. (Pick the leaves from the mid-rib and wash them well.) Slice the onion and potato and fry gently in the butter until they are soft.

Add the dandelion leaves and then stir in the stock and simmer for about twenty minutes. Put the soup through a sieve or liquidise it, then serve hot with wholemeal bread.

Dandelion salad
For this famous French salad blanch the plants by putting an upturned bucket over them for some weeks until the leaves have a mild taste. Then slice cooked beetroot, mix it with chopped dandelion leaves and sprinkle with vinaigrette salad dressing.

Dandelion as vegetable
Strip the leaves from the bitter mid-rib and simmer in boiling water for about ten minutes, then drain and toss in melted butter. They are very good with bacon or ham and are often made up early in the year when 'greens' are scarce.

Dandelion beer
Take 450 g (1 lb) of dandelion plants, including the roots, 450 g (1 lb) of sugar, 4.5 litres (1 gallon) of water, 30 g (1 oz) each of yeast, cream of tartar and sliced ginger root. Boil the dandelion and the ginger in the water for ten minutes. Strain and add the sugar and cream of tartar. Allow to cool to room temperature and then add the

yeast. Cover and leave for three days, then bottle and store in a cool place for a week, when it will be ready to use.

ELDER —
Sambucus nigra
Parts used: Bark, leaves, flowers, berries

The legends that cling to the elder tree are too many to relate. Judas is said to have hanged himself from the elder. The Cross of Calvary is reputed to have been made from an elder tree. And in early pagan Europe the elder was associated with magic and even, in Denmark, dwelt in by the Elder-tree Mother. In many countries it was invested in the people's minds with the power to protect them from evil and black magic.

The incredible number of cures and benefits to man which come from this tree probably accounts for the awe in which it was held in less sceptical and less scientific times than our own. There is space here to mention only a few of them.

Apart from its uses in the manufacture of shoemakers' pegs, needles for weaving nets and an endless collection of handy implements, the elder provides a formidable collection of medicinal remedies. The leaves, bruised and worn about the person, will ward off unwelcome insects in hot weather. The bark is a most effective purgative when decocted. An ointment made from the green inner bark is an instant cure for burns, and one made from the leaves is a useful antidote to sprains, bruises and wounds. The leaves, boiled until soft with a little linseed oil, make an application for piles. The green leaves, heated and applied to the head, are reputed to cure headache. Elderflower water, used in skin and eye lotions, is difficult to make as the flowers have to be expertly saved and dried, but try this recipe for skin beauty from your grandmother's time. Fill a big jar with elderblossoms (no stalks). Compress the blossoms, pour on 2.3 litres (2 quarts) of boiling water and very shortly add 40 ml (1½ fl oz) of rectified spirits. Cover with a cloth, allow to stand till cold, then strain through muslin. Seal the container very well.

Elderberry rob, made from the juice of elderberries simmered with sugar, is an ancient and marvellous recipe for holding off coughs and colds. Dilute a tablespoonful in a mug of hot water for that winter nightcap and go to bed warm and fortified against the chills of the dark season.

Herb as food

Pickled elder shoots

This eighteenth-century recipe has stood the test of time. Pick the young green shoots and cut them with a sharp knife, discarding any tough or woody parts. Peel them carefully, put into a bowl of salted water and leave overnight. Next day combine in a saucepan 600 ml (1 pint) of white wine vinegar, a half-teaspoon of white pepper, a teaspoon of black pepper, three or four blades of mace, a half-teaspoon of ground allspice and one teaspoon of ground ginger. Simmer all these ingredients together for quarter of an hour. Drain the elder shoots, rinse them and pack them into warm dry jars, then strain the hot pickling liquid over them and cover loosely. Sterilise the jars of pickled elder shoots before tightening the lids and storing.

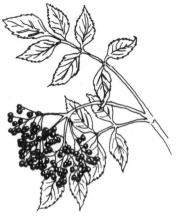

Elderberry

Elderflower fritters

Pick elderflowers and remove from the stalks leaving a short bit of stem attached to each cluster. To make the batter, combine in a bowl 110 g (4 oz) of flour with 150 ml (¼ pint) of lukewarm water, one tablespoonful of liquid honey and two tablespoonfuls of best salad oil. Mix well with a wooden spoon until the batter is smooth. Just before using it beat up the whites of two eggs stiffly and fold into the batter. Pour some oil into a pan to a depth of half an inch. Heat the oil, dip each flowerhead into the batter and shake off any surplus, then lay the flowers flat-side downwards in the hot fat. When cooked turn them over and cook on the other side. Drain on kitchen paper and serve dusted with caster sugar and lemon.

Elderflower champagne

Gather 600 ml (1 pint) of elderflowers snipped from their stems. Slice one lemon and put it with the flowers and 450 g (1 lb) of sugar in a plastic bucket or large bowl. Bring 4.5 litres (1 gallon) of water to the boil, allow it to cool and pour it over the flowers and sugar in the bucket. Stir thoroughly with a wooden spoon, cover and leave for three days. Strain and pour the liquid into clean dry bottles with screw-on caps. It will be ready to drink within three to four weeks but it is best kept for about six months.

Elderberry rob

An ancient cure for colds and sore throats, taken two tablespoonfuls to a mug of boiling water, elderberry rob can also serve as a refreshing drink if mixed with a little soda water and a strong dash of lemon juice. It can be used as a sauce or flavouring for ice cream or yoghurt. Draw the stalks of ripe elderberries through the prongs of a fork and collect the berries in a saucepan. Cover them with water and simmer gently, crushing them the while with the back of a wooden spoon. Strain through a jelly-bag and allow to drip overnight. Stir in 450 g (1 lb) of sugar to every 600 ml (1 pint) of juice. Heat gently, stirring all the time until the sugar has dissolved, then boil for about ten minutes until thick and syrupy. Skim, pour into clean bottles and cork tightly.

EUCALYPTUS —
Eucalyptus globulus
Part used: The oil of the leaves

A native of Australia, this tree comes in a large number of species, grows to a great height and produces prodigious quantities of medicinal, aromatic and industrial oils. One of the species, the *Eucalyptus amygdalin*, is the tallest tree in the world, even taller than the Californian Big Tree (*Sequoia gigantea*), reaching to nearly 150 metres (500 feet). Among its many benefits is its ability to soak up water from fever-laden marshes and simultaneously kill the various creatures which breed malaria and other diseases by its powerful antiseptic exhalations. The wettest, most unhealthy part of Algiers was very quickly converted into the driest and healthiest through the introduction of the eucalyptus tree in the later nineteenth century.

The medicinal eucalyptus oil is obtained by aqueous distillation of the fresh leaves of the *Eucalyptus globulus*. It is readily available from chemists and is a most potent antiseptic. It can be used, well diluted, as a gargle. It is anti-malarial and in spasmodic throat problems it can be applied externally. The oil is useful in the sterilisation of medical instruments. It is sometimes administered in small doses, taken internally, for tuberculosis and other diseases of the lung, but this should be done only under strict medical supervision as larger doses can cause malfunction of the kidneys and even lead to respiratory failure. The oil is useful for inhalation for asthma, colds and sinusitis. It also acts as a disinfectant for cuts and sores. It is important to realise that this most powerful of nature's antiseptics should be treated with respect and not too liberally applied in any case. With eucalyptus it is more than usually true that a little goes a long way.

EYEBRIGHT —
Euphrasia officinalis
Part used: Herb

This little plant with its tiny white or lilac-coloured flowers belongs to that collection of herbs whose names give immediate witness to their medicinal virtues, names like the pilewort (or lesser celandine), the feverfew, and the knitbone (or comfrey). The reputation of the eyebright rests on its ability to bring relief to eyes which have become sore for various reasons. Six hundred years ago it was already established as a herb to cure all complaints of the eye. In the time of Queen Elizabeth I there was an 'Eyebright Ale'; whether the herb was an ingredient is not known, but it is certainly possible.

The eyebright has been credited with helping the memory as well as the sight. A lotion of this herb made with the herb golden seal is considered very effective against disorders of the eye. The juice expressed from the fresh plant is sometimes used or an infusion in milk, though the infusion in water is most commonly applied. When the eyes are very painful, a warm, though not hot, infusion is used; otherwise the remedy is applied cold. But the eyebright has a further use of recent discovery which is that it controls attacks of hay fever and heavy colds if a weakened infusion is administered to the nose and the higher part of the throat every couple of hours. This is really not so surprising when we realise that the mucous membrane or inner skin runs from the eyes right through the body as a kind of moist lining. It seems to follow that whatever affects the lining of the eyelids may also affect the nose, throat and mouth, etc.

FENNEL —
Foeniculum vulgare
Parts used: Seeds, leaves, roots

The fennel is a splendidly graceful, voluminous and immensely healthy green plant that will thrive almost anywhere and can be eaten as a vegetable or used to garnish fish. It was cultivated in ancient times for its seeds and shoots, which are delightful to eat, and its medicinal capacities, as well as for its ornamental character.

Fennel has long enjoyed the reputation of being good for the sight. Even serpents were said to eat fennel and rub their eyes in it to improve their vision. The seed of the fennel is used with purgatives to prevent gripe in the patient. An infusion of the seed or of the leaves is most immediately beneficial for flatulence or indeed for any digestive upset. It is particularly helpful on those occasions in our lives when, whether inadvertently or not, we have overindulged and are beginning to pay the inevitable price. Fennel has similar properties to dill, which is the major ingredient in the well-known gripe-water for infants. Syrup made from juice of the fennel was once given for chronic coughs. Nursing mothers will have more, and more wholesome, milk if they boil the leaves or the seeds in barley water and drink this liquid. For those who are worried about being over their desired weight level, fennel taken in any of its various preparations has a well-established record for reducing the figure to presentable proportions.

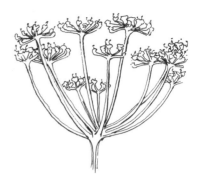

Fennel

Herb as food

In former times fennel was sold by fishmongers for a sauce to accompany fish meals as an aid to digestion. The sauce is made by removing the fennel leaves from the stems and chopping them up very fine. Then a white sauce is prepared and the chopped fennel leaves are stirred in until the sauce turns a deep green. This sauce is good with all fish dishes, but especially with the oily ones such as mackerel. A quicker version is made with a carton of thick cream and lemon juice to taste. Whip the cream, stir in the lemon juice and then the chopped fennel leaves. This sauce is also delicious with roast pork chops.

Another piquant sauce to serve with mackerel is made with 225 g (½ lb) of green gooseberries cooked gently in a saucepan with two tablespoonfuls of water. Simmer gently until the gooseberries are soft and then rub them through a sieve. Return the gooseberries to the pan and add 30 g (1 oz) of butter and one tablespoon of finely chopped fennel leaves. Heat the sauce and serve; or pour the sauce over the cooked fish and heat under the grill for a few minutes before serving.

FEVERFEW —
Chrysanthemum parthenium
Part used: Herb

The name gives us the clue to the main medical application of this herb. A common plant, growing in the shelter of hedges, it has a strong and bitter smell and is avoided by bees. It is popular among country folk, however, who know it to be a powerful antidote to fevers from whatever source.

Feverfew is a general tonic and helps people over nervousness, hysteria and general debility of mind and spirit. An infusion of the herb will assist greatly in these cases. A decoction, possibly made with honey, will help to dispel coughs and colds. A tincture of the herb relieves insect bites of various kinds and a diluted tincture, rubbed all over the body, will ward off predatory insects on hot and humid days. It is said to have a purifying effect on air and atmosphere and is sometimes planted around dwelling places in the hope that it will keep diseases and fevers at bay. In recent times feverfew has been found to be most helpful to people suffering from migraine. A few leaves of the herb taken in a sandwich or tablets (easily available from chemists and health food shops) are the simplest means of benefiting from this particular blessing. Feverfew once had the reputation of being an effective antidote to an excess of opium; if this proved true, something worthwhile might be done to assist opium addicts. A related question naturally arises here: are some, any or all of our young drug addicts searching frantically for some simple substance or substances which their systems really and desperately require and which could be adequately supplied by some harmless herb? It is not impossible.

FLAX —
Linum usitatissimum
Part used: Seed

Flax was cultivated in prehistoric times. The making of linen from the flax was known to our remote ancestors before records were kept, even before languages were written down. The seed of the flax, known as linseed, was, and is, the part mainly used for medicinal purposes. The flax is a rather delicately handsome plant with blue blossoms. The seeds ripen when the plant has been harvested if they are given a little time. The ever-thrifty Dutch stack the plants after they pull them, allow a little time for the seeds to ripen, and then reap two harvests in one.

Dutch linseed is in demand

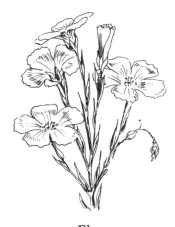

Flax

for medicinal purposes because it is free of contaminants. The oil of the linseed is acquired by expression. The 'cake' which results from this process is valuable forage for cattle or horses. Ground up it becomes known as linseed meal and is used in poultices. These poultices, with

the addition of a little powdered lobelia seeds, relieve pain and discomfort in ulcers, inflammations and boils. Linseed tea can be taken with profit for coughs and colds. This tea, made more palatable by a flavouring of honey, should be taken in wine-glassful amounts. The seeds, which can be purchased at health food shops, bring relief from constipation when swallowed with a glass of water. Linseed tea can be taken for irritation of the urinary organs. Linseed oil, mixed in equal amounts with lime water, is a most effective cure for scalds and burns. Only linseed oil purchased from a chemist should be used; the linseed oil from paint shops is not suitable for medicinal purposes.

GARLIC —
Allium sativum
Part used: Bulb

Garlic has been cultivated by man for so long that it is not possible to say where it came from. The most likely origin is somewhere in southern Asia. Cheops, one of the pharaohs of ancient Egypt, caused pieces of garlic to be distributed daily to his workmen to give them strength to build the Great Pyramid; it has remained a favourite health-giving herb ever since. So what is so wonderful about this strong-smelling cousin of the ordinary onion (or, as the Greeks call it, the 'stinking rose')?

Well, simply that it has spectacular healing powers. During the First World War there was a huge demand for garlic as an antiseptic. The raw juice was squeezed out and diluted with distilled water; swabs of sphagnum moss were dipped in the resulting liquid and applied to the open wound. Given the horrendous destruction of body and limb then in progress, garlic must have been effective, for it would have been abandoned very quickly if it had not been doing its antiseptic job. An unpeeled clove of garlic kept in the mouth for as long as you can bear it does wonders for blocked sinuses and general oral hygiene. Don't be tempted to bite it, though, or you'll burn your mouth badly. Garlic was once used to cure leprosy and smallpox. A syrup of garlic is very good for asthma, coughs, laboured breathing and for most problems of the lungs. Garlic is good for rheumatism, for all infectious diseases — in fact for almost everything. Don't give it to sufferers from skin diseases, however, or to nursing mothers, for it will taint the milk and give colic to the infant. Too much garlic can also irritate the kidneys.

The antiseptic qualities of garlic make it a herb which prevents as well as cures diseases. For this reason it is good to take garlic in food as it helps greatly in the efforts of the system to overcome the various impurities which are part and parcel of the food we eat and, indeed, of the very air we breathe. Even a short list of the ailments for which garlic provides a cheap and effective remedy makes impressive reading.

With hypertension the herb works by opening the blood vessels, thereby bringing down the blood pressure and taking strain off the heart. The relief thus achieved enables the patient to return to a more normal and active routine of life without the side-effects which are such a drawback in conventional drug treatments. Asthma and bronchitis both gain considerable relief from garlic in whatever form it is taken. Its antiseptic qualities, including its extremely strong smell, are first-class germ-killers. It is well worth bearing with the smell to enjoy the relief brought by the natural oil to infected sinus and bronchi. The digestive tract also benefits greatly from the taking of garlic in any of its many forms. It reduces the number of unfriendly bacteria and increases the number of friendly ones.

This aids the processes of digestion and enables us to take more nourishment from the food we eat. Painful joints can be rubbed with garlic and even pimples disappear if rubbed. But in both cases the garlic should also be taken internally to aid the elimination of the residues which tend to cause these complaints to begin with. In the days before penicillin, garlic was a main treatment for tuberculosis, achieving many notable successes.

There are some people who, with the best will in the world, find this marvellous herb difficult, or even impossible, to take. This difficulty can be overcome by taking capsules of it called 'perles' which slip down easily and leave much less taste or smell on the breath. You might also try introducing a very little garlic in food and increasing the amount slightly over a long period; its considerable beneficial effect on the digestion should help to make it acceptable over time. The destruction of intestinal worms is not the least of garlic's services to man and it may be that your system's initial resistance to it is related to the presence of such parasites. But it is worth taking even a small amount of garlic from time to time as a form of insurance against a wide variety of illnesses.

The peoples of the Mediterranean lands take a great deal of garlic in food and even as a casual 'chew' in the same way as certain people in the US, and more recently in Europe, take chewing-gum. Apart from the fact that garlic can't be stuck on the undersides of café tables, there is no comparison between the benefits it confers and those (if any) of the offending 'gum'. It is reported that the garlic-eating peoples are healthier than their non-garlic-eating relatives of the north. Perhaps children should be introduced to the herb at an early age, though how this could safely be done is a matter for further thought, as you will soon discover if you try to chew a piece yourself. The oil of garlic is strong stuff and will burn the mouth of the uninitiated. So if you are introducing it — either to yourself or your children — exercise extreme caution.

Herb as food

Garlic is the key to fine flavouring in cooking, for it has the virtue of releasing and enhancing all the other flavours inherent in the dish. However, a very little of garlic goes a very long way, such is its power to permeate all foods with which it comes in contact. The French speak of a point of garlic, by which they mean the very smallest amount that can be taken on the point of a knife, and the French both love and understand the herb. To introduce garlic into salads, they soak small pieces of bread in a little olive oil mixed with garlic oil, place them in the bottom of the salad bowl, put the salad on top and allow the aroma of the garlic to permeate the salad for about a quarter of an hour. They then remove the bread and toss the salad. The bread, which is no longer part of the salad and is sometimes simply put aside, makes delicious eating for garlic lovers.

Perhaps the best and easiest way to introduce garlic into the diet is to rub a cut clove about the insides of cooking utensils and salad bowls. Once the family has become accustomed to the aroma and taste of garlic and has even begun to expect its strong presence, you might squeeze a clove either over a fairly large salad or into a stew or soup. A special garlic press can be acquired cheaply at any kitchen utensil shop.

To tenderise and enhance the flavour of meat, make a few slits in it near the bone and slip a clove of garlic into each. The number of cloves depends on the weight of the joint and on your own taste; after a little experience you will know how much to use. Any meat, beef

steak in particular, can be rubbed with the cut side of a clove of garlic before cooking.

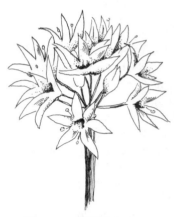

Ramsons (Wild Garlic)

Garlic butter

Peel eight cloves of garlic and crush them together with 225 g (½ lb) of butter. There is of course quite a variation in the size of garlic cloves. This mixture, even with moderately sized cloves, can be very powerful. It is probably best to make your first garlic butter at the rate of two cloves to 225 g (½ lb) of butter and then increase the amount of garlic to taste.

Garlic loaf

Take a light loaf of French bread and cut into slices, leaving the bottom crust intact. Butter the slices on both sides with the garlic butter, then press the loaf together again.

Wrap and bake in a hot oven for ten minutes or to taste. Serve immediately.

Garlic purée
This can be served as a sauce with savoury dishes. Blanch several cloves of garlic, then cook them in butter or oil until soft. Add one dessertspoonful of thick white sauce for each clove. Blend and sieve and serve hot.

Cold garlic sauce
Blanch cloves of garlic, then cook them gently in butter or olive oil until soft. Beat the garlic with a wooden spoon until smooth and add mayonnaise to taste. This sauce is especially good with hard-boiled eggs, cold chicken or cold fish.

Garlic omelette
Take two slices of dry bread, one large clove of garlic, 55 g (2 oz) of butter, four eggs and one dessertspoonful of chopped parsley. Trim the crusts off the bread and cut each slice into small cubes. Peel and crush the garlic. Heat the butter in a frying pan leaving just enough aside to cook the omelette, and fry the bread until golden, stirring constantly and adding the crushed garlic. Remove from the pan and set aside. Break the eggs into a bowl and beat lightly. Heat the remaining butter in the pan and add the eggs. As the eggs start to cook, add the garlic-flavoured cubes of bread and continue to cook. Serve on a hot dish with the parsley sprinkled over the omelette.

Garlic vinegar
Take one clove of garlic, ten tablespoons of basil and 600 ml (1 pint) of white wine vinegar. Peel and crush the garlic and add it to the chopped basil leaves. Bring 300 ml (½ pint) of the vinegar to the boil and add to the garlic and basil leaves, pounding them well together. Leave to cool and then add the remaining vinegar and pour into a jar. Cover and leave for about two weeks stirring occasionally, then strain and bottle.

GOLDEN ROD —
Solidago virgaurea
Parts used: Flowers

This tall woody plant with its crown of golden flowers is familiar to gardeners everywhere. It grows easily in most locations and will spread quickly if not checked. The part which is used medicinally is the flowering tip, picked in July and dried away from the sun. Extremely useful as a diuretic, it easily rids the system of bile and is also effective in strengthening the capillaries against haemorrhaging. It can be applied to bruises and wounds and has the reputation of being extraordinarily effective in removing stones from the urinary tract. Golden rod is known to alleviate rheumatism and can remedy internal ulcers. The usual means of administration is by infusion. Decoctions are the standard means of applying the herb externally. These decoctions can be used to soak swabs for the treatment of cuts and wounds. Golden rod is used in homoeopathic medicine, which employs fasting and simple eating as part of a process of eliminating waste material from the body. Golden rod stimulates the kidneys and the liver, which assist in the expulsion of unwanted substances, thereby invigorating the entire system. The importance of keeping the body free from toxic wastes can be understood from the efforts made by so many herbs to speed up their expulsion. The retention in the system for comparatively long periods of the waste from red meat is increasingly being blamed for bowel cancers.

HAWTHORN —
Crataegus oxyacantha
Parts used: Leaves, fruit

From prehistoric times the hawthorn has been the universal emblem of protection against evil. The early Greeks brought sprigs of thorn to weddings as tokens of the prosperity and joy they wished for the bride and groom. The 'burning bush' of the biblical story of Moses was a species of hawthorn. In early Christian times the hawthorn was revered for being the supposed timber from which Christ's crown of thorns was made. Evidence for the persistence of this belief is found in John McCormack's famous 'Fairy Tree' song.

It is small wonder that the hawthorn was anciently thought to be magical. For though our remote ancestors might not have been as scientifically aware in certain matters as we are (or think we are), they did know that the hawthorn brought relief for vertigo, pleurisy, insomnia and gout; that it was a most effective agent for the regulation of arterial blood pressure as well as being a stimulant to the heart, acting as a sedative upon the cardio-vascular system and benefiting angina pectoris and palpitations. If your nervous system is feeling frayed and fragile, you could not do better than to take an infusion of hawthorn leaves or flowers. This infusion is recommended for those in the early stages of angina, the development of which it is thought to arrest. A decoction of the berries (or haws) can be taken for diarrhoea and dysentery and for sore throats. A decoction of flowers and berries is a good lotion for facial skin problems, including acne. The hawthorn has fewer toxic substances than most herbs or trees. Mix hawthorn leaves with your ordinary Indian tea; they counteract the ingredient in the tea that drives up the blood pressure, and improve the taste. How much more magical could any tree or herb be? Warning: benign as the hawthorn undoubtedly is, it may interact with powerful modern drug preparations. Consult your professional practitioner.

Herb as food
Hawthorn leaf tea
Gather young hawthorn leaves on dry spring days; lay them in a single layer on cardboard in an airing cupboard or over a boiler for three days. Shred and store them in airtight jars away from the light.

Hawthorn flower syrup
Pick 1.1 litres (2 pints) of hawthorn flowers. Pack the freshly picked flower sprays into jars in layers one inch thick with a sprinkling of caster sugar between each two layers. Put 900 g (2 lbs) of sugar in a saucepan with 1.1 litres (2 pints) of water and the strained juice of two lemons. Heat over a low fire until the sugar has dissolved, then boil for three minutes, set aside to cool and stir in five tablespoons of rosewater. Pour the cooled syrup into the jars of hawthorn flowers, screw the lids on loosely and sterilise them in a pot of simmering water for one hour. Take the jars out of the water and when quite cold strain the syrup into small bottles. Store the syrup in a cool place.

Haw jelly
The berries from different hawthorn trees vary greatly in size. Pick the larger ones in the autumn and remove the stalks. Put into a saucepan and just cover them with cold water. Bring to the boil and simmer until very soft, crushing the haws from time to time with the back of a wooden spoon. Strain overnight through a jelly-bag and the next day measure the resulting liquid. To every 600 ml (1 pint) of liquid add 450 g (1 lb) of sugar and the strained juice of two lemons. Put into a large saucepan and heat gently, stirring all the time until the sugar has dissolved. Then boil rapidly until the jelly sets when tested on a cold plate. Pour into clean, warm jars. Cover and store.

HOLLY —
Ilex aquifolium
Parts used: Leaves, berries, bark

Holly is always green and, like other evergreens, over the centuries it came to be considered an emblem of good fortune. It is, of course, above all associated with the feast of Christmas. There is a legend that holly first sprang up in the footprints of Christ and that its red berries and prickly leaves represent Christ's sufferings. In some European countries the holly is still called Christ's Thorn or the Holy Tree.

Very few insects live around the holly. Sheep thrive on holly leaves. The berries are eaten voraciously by birds with no apparent ill effects, but they are violently purgative to humans and children should be made aware of their dangers. An infusion of holly leaves was once prescribed for catarrh and smallpox. The leaves are febrifuge and a decoction helps patients with influenza, pneumonia and bronchitis by ridding the body of the waste matter associated with these ailments. Sweeten the decoction with a little honey as it is very sour to taste. The berries and bark made useful fomentations for broken bones in olden days. The expressed juice of the fresh leaves has been used to remedy jaundice. The only comparatively safe application for the berries is to dry and powder them, then sprinkle on serious cuts to stop bleeding. If you need to cut holly back in the autumn when it has berries on it, or if the birds are feasting on the berries and you fear there will be none left for Christmas, stick the twigs you cut in the earthen floor of a garden shed. The berries will remain fresh well into the new year.

HOLLY, SEA —
Eringium maritinum
Part used: Root

This prickly plant, which looks like a thistle, is found growing by the sea-shore but will also grow inland and was once a favourite in ornamental gardens. The flowers, leaves and roots may be eaten and are all very nourishing. The roots in particular are very popular in some countries and are alleged to have aphrodisiac qualities. They were available in a candied form in sweet shops not too long ago. It was an ancient remedy for people who were withered with age and in want of natural moisture. The best specimens of sea holly are found on the sandy sea-shore, where they have access to salt water.

The dried roots are of great value with coughs that have become chronic. Persistent nervous ailments and nervous conditions brought on by other illnesses all improve upon the taking of the sea holly root. A decoction of the root is very stimulating to the action of the kidneys and bladder; it can be taken in whatever quantity the patient thinks appropriate. The roots also have a reputation, when bruised and boiled in lard, of being of singular use when applied to broken bones and also of actually helping flesh to replace itself where some has been removed. If you should decide to bring the sea holly on from seed, remember to sow it in autumn; otherwise it may not germinate. Sow it in the sun, which it prefers, being a native of the open sea-shore.

HOPS —
Humulus lupulus
Parts used: Flowers, fruit, leaves

A relation of the stinging nettle, the hop grows wild in Britain but is not a native of Ireland. Its principal and best-known use is in the manufacture of beer, but it has many strictly medicinal applications too. Hops are grown on an extensive scale in southern England and in various European countries, in fact in most places where beer and ale are made.

The fruit of the hop, which is cone-shaped, is the part mainly employed for medicinal purposes, helping to restore lost appetite and also to induce sleep. Hops are taken either as an infusion or as a tincture. Both preparations are believed to bring rest and tranquility to patients who suffer from some nervous complaint or have simply had a traumatic experience. The infusion is most beneficial in cases of heart ailments and is also a remedy for jaundice and indigestion, indeed for all upsets of the liver or stomach. Hop tea, made from the leaves mixed with Indian tea, combines the stimulation of the one with the calming effect of the other. A fomentation of hops, perhaps in combination with camomile, relieves pain and reduces inflammation in cases of boils, bad bruises, rheumatic pains and swellings generally. Hops may also be used to make a poultice; and a pillow of warmed hops has long been employed to relieve toothache, neuralgia, earache and related complaints. Can you wonder that beer is so popular? It is almost medicine, as its devotees have always claimed.

HOREHOUND, WHITE —
Marrubium vulgare
Part used: Herb

This bushy plant was known to the Romans for its medicinal value. It was brought by the ancient Jews to their Passover feasts. Even the priests of Egypt were aware of its health-giving properties. It is found throughout Europe, both cultivated and as an escape from cultivation. It should not be confused with the black horehound.

White horehound is effective as a remedy for diseases of the lung. It was given to ease consumption in years gone by, and asthmatics and others with congested lungs obtain great relief from it. A decoction of the herb combined with rue, liquorice root, marshmallow root and hyssop will work wonders with a chronic cough and even with consumption. Made into a syrup, white horehound is both a tonic and a remedy for coughs in children; it has the added benefit of settling their stomachs. An infusion is adequate for the common cold and will bring ease and a sense of well-being if taken three or four times in the day. The leaves of the white horehound can be dried, powdered and used as a vermifuge while the leaves can also be boiled with lard into an ointment useful for healing cuts and abrasions. Candied horehound, made by boiling the fresh plant and extracting its juices, is an easy means of administering this herb. Large doses of the herb will have a mild laxative effect. White horehound restores appetite, strengthens the heart, helps to remedy malaria and has a tonic effect on the liver.

Herb as food
Horehound candy
For this sweet, traditionally loved by children, assemble 85 g (3 oz) of fresh horehound, two cups of water, 900 g (2 lbs) of brown sugar and a quarter-cup of corn syrup. Cook the horehound slowly in water for quarter of an hour in a heavy saucepan. Let it stand for an hour. Strain and add the sugar and syrup to the liquid and heat gently until the sugar dissolves. Then boil until it sets hard when a little is dropped into a cup of cold water. Pour into a greased pan and mark into squares.

Horehound beer
Add a cupful of leaves and stems to 13.5 litres (3 gallons) of water and 900 g (2 lbs) of treacle. Simmer for an hour, then strain and cool to room temperature. Add two tablespoonfuls of yeast, cover with a clean

cloth and allow to stand until the following day. Strain and bottle. It will be ready for drinking in one week.

HORSERADISH —
Cochlearia armoracia
Part used: Root

Horseradish has been known, both as a condiment and as a source of medicinal assistance, certainly since the early Middle Ages, but probably long before then. We associate it with the taking of red meat, particularly beef, but it is also still used medicinally both in orthodox medicine and in herbal preparations. The root is the only part used now though in earlier times the leaves were also employed for the relief of various ailments.

Horseradish has powerful antiseptic qualities when applied to an external wound. Sufferers from dropsy find it helpful as do those in a mild fever. Two or three tablespoonfuls of a decoction three times a day will relieve the dropsy. Combined with nutmeg, orange peel and spirit of wine, the horseradish corrects a sluggish digestion. Swellings of the joints and general discomfort associated with gout, or even swellings of the liver and spleen, will benefit from an external application of the bruised root. The entire system benefits from horseradish taken in any of the various forms given above. It is an old but tried and true method — thought by some to be the very best — of getting rid of worms in children. In Argentina a large proportion of the adult population suffers from tapeworm, caused by eating beef in excess. If they take horseradish with the beef it will surely overcome the tapeworm.

Herb as food
The roots of the horseradish are grated, ground or minced in a sauce with cream. Its flavour is robust and hot like that of mustard. While its main fame rests on its suitability as an accompaniment to beef, its lesser-known but equally effective use lies in its suitability as a sauce for shellfish dishes. The well-known Hans Andersen sandwich of Denmark consists of bacon and liver pâté garnished with tomato and horseradish taken on rye bread.

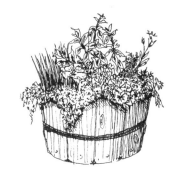

HORSETAIL —
Equisetum arvense
Part used: Herb

The horsetail belongs to a very primitive order of plant, being nearest related to the ferns and descending from the carboniferous period of geo-time. The plant, which reaches about 38 cm (15 inches), looks a bit like a miniature pine tree. It will grow almost anywhere, but especially quickly and plentifully in loose sand if it once gets rooted in it.

Medicinally the horsetail has many functions. It cleans wounds and heals bleeding, and is very effective against kidney and bladder dysfunction, including kidney stone. A cup of horsetail tea a day is a well-tried remedy for the pains of rheumatism and gout; this tea will also stop vomiting of blood and internal haemorrhaging. Difficulty in urinating can be lessened by applying the steam of horsetail (not too hot) to the affected part. Some infections cause retention of water; horsetail tea will release and rid the body of that water. It is known to be effective in cases where several other diuretics have failed. A footwash with a little of decoction of horsetail is most efficacious for cracked feet, athlete's foot and fungal diseases. It is particularly good for sweaty feet. This decoction will also remedy ringworm if rubbed on the offending places. Ringworm is a fungal infection and not a worm under the skin as we all believed when we were children.

HOUSELEEK —
Sempervivum tectorum
Part used: Fresh leaves

This most fascinating plant can be seen on the roofs of houses in the countryside throughout Europe. The Emperor Charlemagne actually ordered that it should be grown on roofs, in the belief that it protected the house against fire and lightning. Like so many ancient customs, there is more to it than meets the eye; quite apart from the fact that the houseleek is singularly adapted to growing on roofs, and that it preserves thatched roofs from decay, it is a living medicine chest in itself.

The Latin name *Sempervivum* means, roughly, 'ever living', and *tectorum* refers to the roof. The sheer health of the houseleek is borne out by its length of life and by the medicinal benefits it confers on the household sensible enough to grow one, either on the roof or on a rough and rocky patch of the garden. The houseleek, through its juice, bestows a cure for burns, ulcers, scalds and many afflictions of the skin. A poultice of the bruised leaves or a compress of the juice will bring quick relief. Even headaches are said to cease when a compress of the expressed juice is placed on the head. Mix the juice with honey and take it for thrush in the mouth. The leaves, like dock leaves, soothe nettle stings and will also help with bee stings. The inner surface of the cut leaves was once used as a remedy for warts. Houseleek spreads quickly, so beware. But if you grow it on your roof and wish it to spread, stick the offsets of the plant to the tiles, slates or whatever material there is with a piece of earth and leave the rest to nature.

HYSSOP —
Hyssopus officinalis
Part used: Herb

Hyssop means the 'holy herb' in Greek. It was used for cleansing temples and shrines, and the Bible mentions it as a purge. A low evergreen shrub, the hyssop is a native of the Mediterranean lands but can be grown in these islands. There are three varieties, known by their flowers, which are white, blue and red. With its splendid aroma, hyssop is used a great deal in the making of liqueurs and is a major ingredient of chartreuse. The aroma is also strongly present in honey made from the hyssop.

Medicinally, the hyssop has many virtues. Mixed with horehound it makes an excellent infusion for worms. Sufferers from asthma do well to boil the green tops in soup, and hyssop tea strengthens the stomach against upsets and nervousness.

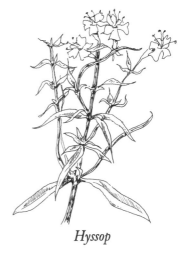

Hyssop

The bruised herb is a great healer of cuts and wounds, and tea made with the fresh green tops is a well-known remedy for rheumatism. An infusion of hyssop encourages expectoration and is most effective in removing catarrh from the chest. Hippocrates gives hyssop as a treatment for pleurisy and bronchitis; other ancient sources recommended that it be boiled with honey to combat various lung complaints.

It is not advisable to take strong decoctions or infusions of hyssop as it can have an irritating effect on anyone with a nervous condition. Again, it must be emphasised that with herbal remedies, less is definitely more; quality is so much more important than quantity. Like all the best medicines of every kind, herbal remedies persuade your system to heal itself.

Herb as food

Hyssop is like a slightly sharply flavoured mint. Its tender tops and leaves are the parts used in cooking and they give life and interest to a range of foods from fruit pies to stews, through fruit cocktails (especially cranberry), oily fish and soups. They also combine well in various stuffings.

Hamburgers with hyssop

Add a dash of interest to hamburgers by including hyssop for flavour. To 450 g (1 lb) of meat add one chopped onion and a finely chopped clove of garlic, one and a half tablespoons of chopped parsley, one and a half tablespoons of hyssop, one teaspoon of chopped marjoram and one large egg. Mix them all together and form into burgers. Roll the burgers in sesame seeds and cook in hot oil. Serve hot.

JUNIPER —
Juniperus communis
Parts used: Ripe fruit (which has been carefully dried), leaves

The juniper is a coniferous tree which reaches a height of only about 1.8 metres (6 feet) in these islands. In classical times its branches were hung above doors and windows as their perfume was thought to repel snakes. During plagues the juniper was burnt in cities and towns for its strong disinfectant power. Juniper berries have many uses in the seasoning of various kinds of fish and fowl and are a main ingredient in gin, to which they lend a fetching aroma.

Many ailments are remedied by the juniper. An infusion of crushed berries will be found helpful in the treatment of urinary tract disorders such as gravel, cystitis, cirrhosis, prostatis and diabetes. It increases the volume of the urine and gives it an odour of violets. This infusion is also recommended for rheumatism and arthritis, bronchial catarrh, general debility and sluggishness, loss of appetite and digestive upset. The berries that survive three years and acquire a kind of blue-black colour are the ones to use; these are eaten with advantage by most animals, sheep being thought to benefit particularly. Caution should be exercised with this infusion; take only 600 ml (1 pint) in twenty-four hours. Excessive doses could cause irritation. Consult your herbalist.

Herb as food
Crushed juniper berries enhance the aroma and flavour of ham, pâté and stuffings for pork, venison and game birds. They add flavour to cabbage, sauerkraut and sauces.

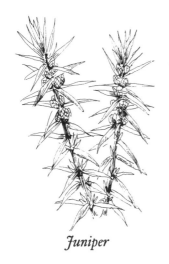

Juniper

Cabbage and juniper
Take 900 g (2 lbs) of white cabbage, one onion finely chopped, one tablespoonful of olive oil, one clove of garlic and ten juniper berries. Shred the cabbage finely, then wash in cold water and drain well. Heat the oil in an ovenproof casserole and gently fry the onion and crushed garlic for a few minutes until they are soft. Stir in the crushed juniper berries, then the shredded cabbage, and season to taste. Cover with a tight-fitting lid and bake in a hot oven for about half an hour until the cabbage is cooked.

Pears in wine with juniper berries
Take three pears, 150 ml (¼ pint) each of red wine and apple juice, two tablespoonfuls of honey, four crushed juniper berries and a quarter-teaspoonful of cinnamon. Peel the pears whole, and mix the red wine, apple juice, honey and juniper berries in a saucepan. Add the pears and simmer for about half an hour, turning the pears in the mixture from time to time. Arrange the pears in a serving dish and pour any remaining syrup over them. Dust with a little cinnamon and serve.

LADY'S MANTLE —
Alchemilla vulgaris
Parts used: Herb, root

As beautiful as its name implies, this herb grows about 30 cm (1 foot) high and is all green, including its flowers. In the Middle Ages it was associated with the Virgin Mary — hence its name. The generic name, *Alchemilla*, comes from the Arabic word for alchemy and refers to the legendary healing powers of this herb., which was once used in magical formulae.

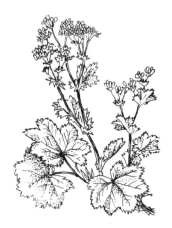

Lady's Mantle

The whole herb — even the root — is used medicinally. It is gathered when in flower in June and July. In olden times the root was given in a decoction, both internally and externally, for wounds and bleedings of all kinds, and was found most efficient in staunching and healing, and in soaking up the moisture associated with wounds. Dried and powdered, the root is excellent for healing wounds and sores. Lady's Mantle is one of several herbs of which it is said that, placed under your pillow at night, it will bring you a good night's sleep. Perhaps it should be called Conscience, or Conscience Ease. Lady's Mantle is mixed with Indian tea

in Switzerland. It is used as a forage plant for cattle with some success; not only does it lead to higher milk yields, but it imparts a most appetising flavour to the cheese made from that milk. However, as grazing animals won't eat the herb until it is saved and fully dry, it is of limited value as a pasture herb.

LAVENDER —
Lavandula vera
Parts used: Flowers, herb

There are many species of this beautifully aromatic herb, but the essential oil of lavender is generally extracted from the *Lavandula vera*. Lavender is of course greatly associated with cosmetics; but part of that association originated in its characteristic of ridding beds and cupboards of bugs, lice and moths — indeed of anything that crawls or flies. Ants, if they find their way to your kitchen press, will be driven off by a few tissues soaked in lavender oil (and by very little else).

Lavender's medicinal applications may appear to have been largely superseded by modern scientific medicine but it is an extremely powerful antiseptic capable, in tiny amounts, of killing various fairly lethal bacilli such as streptococcus, diphtheria and typhoid. The preparations of lavender use the small blue flowers, which are picked before they have quite fully bloomed. An infusion of the herb is good for ailments of the

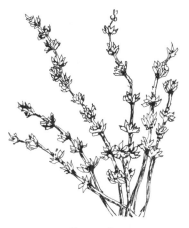

Lavender

nerves like migraines and insomnia. This infusion has a tonic and disinfecting effect and is recommended for problems of the respiratory tract, e.g. laryngitis, asthma and bronchitis, and also for influenza, chills and general feverishness. A tincture of lavender applied as a lotion makes the hair stronger. It is also of use for rubbing on rheumatic joints, while a few drops in a glass of lukewarm water can be very beneficial as a gargle and mouthwash. Lavender oil can remedy scalds and burns , as well as varicose ulcers. Finally, if your dog has fleas and also smells a bit funny,

administer a little lavender oil and kill two birds with one stone.

Herb as food
Lavender sugar
For a delightfully perfumed topping for cakes or biscuits, place equal amounts of bruised fresh lavender flowers and sugar in a jar, put a tight cork on it and shake well every few days. After three weeks sift the sugar and store it for future use.

LOOSESTRIFE, PURPLE —
Lythrum salicaria
Parts used: Herb, root

The purple loosestrife is a tall and very striking plant covered with reddish-purple flowers. It likes to grow in wet places, sometimes in large colonies — one of the more dramatic sights of summer is the loosestrife on display in such strength. Among its non-medical uses in the past was the tanning of leather.

A decoction of purple loosestrife is effective against dysentery. It is also a remedy for fevers, liver diseases and constipation. As a gargle it is good for tonsillitis. The decoction is used to cure sore eyes, in which connection some herbalists consider it superior to the eyebright. An ointment can be made by adding two parts of May butter without salt, two parts of sugar and two parts of wax to one part of the decoction; this cures ulcers and sores. The decoction can be applied externally to sores and cuts, and used in compresses for skin ailments such as eczema and itchy irritations.

There are, of course, several herbal remedies for itches, but the most important thing to remember is not to scratch them. Severe scratching breaks the skin and can give rise to sores and even ulcers. There is a type of soft brush, available commercially, which can be used to ease the itch.

LOVAGE —
Levisticum officinale
Parts used: Root, seeds, leaves and young stems

Lovage is a gentle, humble herb that was never dedicated to gods or saints, was never an official remedy and never had great claims made for its medicinal magic. In other words, it is a cottage plant, grown as a sweet herb. Nevertheless, it has considerable medicinal virtues that are none the worse for being of a mild, ameliorative character.

Lovage, precisely because it is so gentle, is of especial use for remedying flatulence and other disturbances of the digestion in children. It encourages perspiration where such encouragement is required. For all these purposes it can be taken as an infusion of the roots and fruit. Urinary troubles, gravel and jaundice are alleviated by an infusion of the roots. Seeds and roots were once thought beneficial in plague. The root of a related Chinese herb called Kao-Pau is a very effective expectorant; lovage probably has this virtue in a less spectacular form and might be employed to dislodge persistent catarrh. An infusion of the seeds of lovage used cold is an old recipe for clearing up inflammation and general irritation in the eyes. A decoction makes a good throat gargle, especially for quinsy. The leafstalks and stem bases were once eaten, blanched; no doubt this taste will be rediscovered in time, but in the meantime the fact that lovage can be taken as a vegetable proves how safe it is to use as a herb.

Herb as food
Lovage tastes like a rather strong variety of celery. Its stems can be used like celery and they can also be candied like angelica. If you are using lovage to replace celery in stews, salads or soups, a little of

the leaves will achieve the desired effect.

Lovage and tomato soup
Take 110 g (4 oz) of chopped lovage leaves, one chopped onion, 450 g (1 lb) of tomatoes peeled and chopped, 30 g (1 oz) of butter and 900 ml (1½ pints) of chicken stock. Melt the butter in a saucepan and gently cook the onion until soft. Gradually add the rest of the ingredients, stirring all the time. Bring to the boil and simmer for quarter of an hour. Liquidise until smooth and heat through before serving.

MALLOW, MARSH —
Althaea officinalis
Parts used: Leaves, flowers, fruit and root

There are anything up to a thousand species of mallow, few of them having any unwholesome elements from a human point of view. The marshmallow sweet has no connection of any kind with the herb, being made with sugar and gum arabic and eggs; why it should be called by the herb's name is a question you will have to pursue with the manufacturers. The real herbal marsh mallow was considered a great delicacy by the ancient Romans. It is a decorative plant when placed in the right area of the garden.

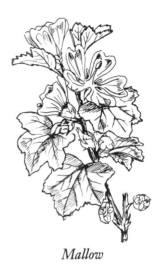

Mallow

All parts of the plant are used in the healing arts. Its main action is a soothing one and it is a very appropriate herb for taking internally, particularly for irritating coughs, colds, laryngitis, constipation, cystitis and catarrhal conditions of the bladder; it can be taken for any of these ailments either as an infusion or as a decoction. A decoction is taken as a gargle for gingivitis, dental abscesses and other conditions of the mouth. The decoction should be inhaled hot with a towel over your head to ease congestion in the sinuses. Teething infants obtain great relief by sucking on a marsh mallow root, a safe means of bringing comfort to their sore gums. The fresh roots of marsh mallow when crushed make a most comforting poultice for inflammations. A syrup made from the marsh mallow is the most suitable way of treating children.

Herb as food

Mallow leaves make one of the best green vegetables of any of the wild plants. Pick young leaves when the plant is in flower and wash them well in cold water. Put the leaves into a pan of boiling water and cook for a few minutes until just tender, being careful not to overcook them. Drain and toss in melted butter.

Mallow soup

Pick 1.1 litres (2 pints) of young mallow leaves, wash well in cold water and shred them. Peel and crush one clove of garlic and fry it gently in a pan with a little butter until it is soft. Add the mallow leaves and pour on 1.1 litres (2 pints) of chicken stock. Simmer the soup for ten minutes and serve with fried bread croûtons floating on the top.

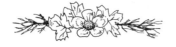

MARIGOLD —
Calendula officinalis
Parts used: Leaves, flowers and herb

The lovely golden flower of the marigold is known to all of us as a garden flower. It has the unusual characteristic of closing early in the afternoon. The flowers are dried and used in broths and are said to bring great ease to the spirits. They were at one time used to colour cheese, and to dye the hair yellow or blonde. Though natives of the Mediterranean lands, marigolds take easily to conditions in our cooler climes. They seed themselves and will scatter quite widely given half a chance.

Medicinal uses include helping chronic ulcers and varicose veins; the flowers are dried away from direct sunlight and are usually given in an infusion. The marigold has the reputation of remedying bee and wasp stings; this sounds a little unlikely, though given the comprehensive chemical make-up of all herbs it is not impossible. The wasp's sting being alkaline, a compress of the acid cider vinegar is most effective as it restores the acid/alkaline balance at the point of the sting; the bee's sting, on the contrary, is acid and therefore the alkaline bicarbonate of soda should be used.

A lotion made from the flower of the marigold gives ease to sore eyes. Marigold tea can be beneficial in cases of diarrhoea. A decoction of the flowers brings out smallpox and measles (the use of marigold in many children's illnesses is an indication of its 'user-friendliness').The marigold is a good example of a plant which is both a pot herb and a medicinal herb. All pot herbs or flavouring herbs yield their medicinal qualities when taken in food and a knowledge of these qualities should help anyone catering for a family to choose whichever herbs fulfil medical as well as gastronomical requirements.

MARJORAM, SWEET —
Origanum marjorana
Parts used: Herb, leaves

Both the cultivated or sweet marjoram and the wild marjoram have the same properties, medicinally speaking. Sweet marjoram is a tall-growing plant with many flowers which are in close heads like knots — hence its nickname, the Knotted Marjoram. It grows well in sandy soil but, being a native of Portugal, will not survive hard weather and must be sown every year. The Greeks used the wild marjoram as an antidote to poisons; they also believed the dead were happy if it grew on their graves. Marjoram is still gathered for tea in the southern counties of England.

The oil of the marjoram, attained by distilling, is potently caustic and should be used with extreme care. The practice of placing a few drops on cotton wool in the cavity of a painful tooth must surely have been made unnecessary by modern dentistry and all its medications. An infusion of the flowering tips is of especial assistance in bringing out measles. An unguent of marjoram, made from the fresh-picked herb, is an effective treatment for rheumatic and muscular aches and pains, being massaged into the affected area. This unguent can be laid on the forehead to ease headaches and on the nose to remedy colds. A poultice placed on stiff parts of the body can bring relief. The powdered herb can be used as a sneezing powder, rather as snuff is used, to clear blocked nasal passages and sinuses. Care should be exercised here as the idea is simply to prompt the reaction of sneezing, and a very little of snuff, marjoram or even dust will achieve that purpose.

Herb as food

Marjoram adds a spicy kind of sweetness to a very broad range of foods. The leaves can be used to advantage with all meat dishes and stews. They can also be used in stuffings, in cooking poultry and with vegetables, especially celery, runner beans, carrot, cabbage and to great effect with potatoes. Salads and soups will gain from marjoram, as will egg, cheese and sauces for fish.

Hot herb cabbage slaw

Shred half a white cabbage. Melt two tablespoonfuls of butter in a large pan and fry the cabbage for several minutes, stirring all the time, then add half a cup of chicken stock with sprigs of fennel and marjoram to taste. Simmer for a few minutes, always stirring, then add half a cup of yoghurt, preferably homemade. Serve in a heated dish.

MEADOWSWEET —
Spiraea ulmaria
Parts used: Herb, flowers

The tall meadowsweet that dominates wet meadows and riverbanks throughout the summer months is one of the best-known and most beloved of wild flowering herbs. Its scent haunts the memory long after summer has faded — or rather its blend of two scents, for an unusual feature of the meadowsweet is that both its flowers and leaves smell distinctly different.

The meadowsweet does not seem to have been used for medicinal purposes until the seventeenth century; but its real moment of glory came in 1853 when Charles Frederic Gerhardt, a chemist in Strasbourg, made from it what became the world's most widely used medication, aspirin. Orthodox medicine depends a great deal on aspirin and in certain situations it has proven its value, but the gentler herbal tablets made from the meadowsweet will in many cases achieve the same end without subjecting the gastric mucosa to the same side-effects. These tablets, readily available in health food and chemists' shops, are beneficial in overcoming influenza and chills, kidney and bladder complaints, dropsy, oedema and gout.

An infusion of the dried herb is of great assistance in cases of diarrhoea among children. It provides nourishment as well as helping to eliminate the problem. An infusion of the fresh flowers brings perspiration in cases of influenza, rather as aspirin does but more gently. It may not be a coincidence that the meadowsweet was one of the three herbs considered most sacred by the ancient druids. (Water-mint and vervain were the other two.)

Herb as food

Stewed apple with meadowsweet

For those who wish to keep their sugar consumption to a minimum this makes the perfect dessert. Surround a muslin bag containing eight or ten flowers of the meadowsweet with about 900 g (2 lbs) of cooking apples which have been peeled and sliced, in a saucepan holding 150 ml (¼ pint) of water. Add one tablespoonful of sugar and simmer slowly for about ten minutes until the apple has softened. Allow to cool in the saucepan, then squeeze the bag of meadowsweet and remove it before serving. Reducing the amount of water makes a similar mixture suitable for filling pies or apple tarts.

NETTLE, COMMON STINGING —
Urtica dioica
Parts used: Leaves, roots

The common nettle is too well known to require detailed description. Its presence usually indicates a soil rich in nitrogen and it is frequently found in the vicinity of human habitation, both ancient and modern.

Up to the end of May, nettles may be gathered and cooked like any other green vegetable and with much greater benefit than many. Wearing rubber gloves, pluck only the four topmost leaves of the young nettles as these are the tenderest and tastiest for cooking, and be sure to pick a good quantity as, like all greens, the nettle tends to diminish in bulk when boiled down. After the beginning of June nettles become too strong for cooking but tea made from the dried nettle (picked in May) can be drunk all the year round, though you must dry it green or it loses its value.

The most important blessing conferred on us by the nettle, especially in the spring, is that it both cleanses and builds our blood, and as our blood is what conditions our entire bodies, all kinds of ailments clear up and we feel new energy coursing through our veins. Take one cup of nettle tea a little while before breakfast and one or two cups during the rest of the day; for maximum effect you should sip and not gulp it down. Never boil the infusion as this destroys its beneficial elements. Too many or too strong infusions of nettle or nettle tea can cause burns all over the body, so if you wish to drink the tea regularly use a light hand with the dried nettle. Using nettle teabags, available in health food shops, relieves you of the bother of saving and drying the nettles and also makes it easier to control the strength of the infusion.

To restore hair growth use a tincture of nettle. Fill a bottle up to the neck with cleaned chopped nettle roots. Pour 40% whiskey or vodka over the roots and leave the bottle standing in a warm place for fourteen days. This tincture should be massaged into the scalp. To make an excellent hair-wash place four or five double-handfuls of nettles (either fresh or dried) in a 5 litre pot (8 ¾ pints), bring to the boil and infuse them for five minutes. A heaped double-handful of roots, soaked in cold water overnight, then boiled and allowed to infuse for ten minutes the following day, will give the same result. Curd soap should be used with the wash in both cases.

Victor Hugo in *Les Misérables* wrote:

Chopped Nettle is good for poultry; pounded Nettle is good for cattle. The Nettle seed mixed with fodder gives a gloss to the coats of animals. The root mixed with salt makes a handsome yellow colour. It makes

first class hay which can be cut twice.

And what does the Nettle require? Little earth, no attention and no cultivation.

Herb as food
Nettle as vegetable
Nettles are a valuable green vegetable in early spring. Gather a basinful of the young tops. Melt one tablespoonful of butter in a saucepan over a low heat and add the washed nettle tops. Cover the saucepan closely and continue cooking very gently for a few minutes until the juice begins to run out of the nettles; you can then increase the heat and simmer for about ten minutes until they are soft. Remove from the heat and put through the liquidiser. Serve hot as a delicious vegetable not unlike spinach.

For thin nettle soup use the above recipe but add chicken stock after the nettles have been liquidised. To make a thick nettle soup, cook diced potato in the chicken stock before adding to the nettle mix.

Nettle pudding
Gather a basinful of young nettle leaves and wash them thoroughly in cold water. Finely slice two onions. Melt a spoonful of butter in a pan and add the nettles, onions and a teaspoonful of chopped marjoram.

Cover the pan and put on a low heat for about five minutes. Grease a pudding bowl and alternate layers of the nettle and of breadcrumbs (110 g/4 oz). Dot with butter and cover the bowl with greaseproof paper, tied down securely. Steam for one hour approx.

OAK, COMMON —
Quercus robur
Parts used: Leaves, bark, gall

If the beech is the queen of the forest, then the oak is the king; and if a mature common oak absorbs the growth potential of ⅓ hectare (⅔ acre), it shelters and sustains a large number of species of insects, plants and parasites. An old name for the oak is 'Tanner's Bark', leather tanners and shoemakers of the past having stripped the oak bark for its tannin content. It is not surprising to learn that these tradesmen were unwelcome guests in forested places. The massive oak roof-frames that survive from the Middle Ages are held together by oak pegs; the tannin in the beams would quickly corrode iron nails.

The same oak bark is now the part of the oak mainly employed in medicine. A decoction treats haemorrhages and, taken with the flowers of the camomile, makes quite a good substitute for quinine. It is useful for piles and to rub on bleeding gums, and as a gargle for sore throat with relaxed uvula. It is sometimes an ingredient in remedies for diarrhoea. A decoction of oak bark and acorns made with milk was once used as an antidote to poisonous herbs. The bruised leaves have a healing effect on wounds.

The oak gall, or so-called 'Oak Apple', is formed from an insect egg out of which emerges a gall-wasp. When the gall is broken open it is found to contain an acidic substance which is used in making ink and dye and also, quite widely, in tanning leather. A tincture of gall is the most powerful of all natural astringents. Tannic acid is very bitter and, taken in quantity, cannot but be harmful to the stomach, however valuable a medicine it can be in extreme cases of dysentery, cholera, etc. Ordinary Indian tea contains tannin.

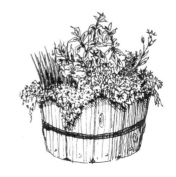

PARSLEY —
Apium petroselinum
Parts used: Roots, seeds, leaves

Not to be confused with fool's parsley, which is poisonous, parsley has a long and distinguished connection with the fortunes of mankind. Homer relates how the chariot horses of his day were given parsley to eat. Parsley was used as a crown for athletes at the Isthmian games in ancient Greece. There was a theory that if you said your enemy's name while pulling up a parsley plant, he would die suddenly. This idea associated parsley with witchcraft and frightened off some people from growing and eating it; but again, as we have seen in the cases of other powerful herbs, this superstition was merely a primitive recognition of the great healing powers of parsley.

Parsley is another example of the combination of pot herb and healing herb, for it is used freely as a pot herb and even as a vegetable; in taking it thus we enjoy its profound medicinal benefits as well as its sheer food value. Parsley is very rich in calcium, iron and various trace elements. Taken in any form it is most beneficial to the kidneys and the urinary tract. It also stimulates blood circulation. A decoction of the dried root is particularly good for sluggishness of the kidney and, as a result, combats gravel, urine retention and arthritis, as well as dropsy and jaundice. A decoction was employed as a remedy for the plague in ancient times. Parsley tea was used successfully during the First World War to treat men in the trenches who had developed kidney complications from dysentery. An infusion of the fresh leaves has a regulatory effect on menstrual discharge and in the process helps to relieve associated pains and cramps.

Herb as food
Some consider parsley to have the widest range of all the culinary herbs. Its flavour is strong but wholesome. The stalks of the parsley are more strongly flavoured than the leaves and are used in stock-pots and stews. The leaves can garnish all manner of vegetable and savoury dishes. They are also taken in cream sauces with omelettes and other egg dishes, in salads and with tongue, ham and fish.

Parsley bread
This is delicious and ideal for a party. Take two tablespoonfuls of chopped parsley, one tablespoonful of chopped chives,

225 g (½ lb) of butter and the juice of a lemon. Beat the herbs into the butter and then add the lemon juice. Mix until very smooth and soft. Slice a loaf of French bread, leaving it attached at the bottom. Spread the slices on both sides with the parsley butter and press the loaf back into shape. For hot bread wrap and bake the loaf in a hot oven before serving.

Green chicken
This recipe is three centuries old. Chop finely a generous bowl of parsley; take four boned and skinned chicken breasts. Dredge with seasoned flour and shake off the excess. Dip into egg and milk, coat with fine breadcrumbs and sauté until cooked. Cool slightly and coat the top side of each piece with beaten egg, then press on a generous amount of the parsley, making sure it sticks well to the chicken. Bake in a warm oven for about ten minutes.

PELLITORY-OF-THE-WALL —
Parietaria officinalis
Part used: Herb

This well-known but unpretentious plant is, as its name indicates, to be found growing on walls and on heaps of broken stone almost every-where. A relative of the stinging nettle and the hop, it is not without its share of medicinal uses. The pellitory grows widely throughout Europe. It thrives in dry places; hence its fondness for walls, whether standing or fallen.

An infusion of the herb is said to be an extremely effective remedy for stone in the bladder, gravel and other urinary complaints. It is best to use this herb fresh as it loses much of its power when dried unless it is dried quickly. An unusual virtue of the pellitory is its ability, when taken as a decoction, to cure a cough which has lasted for a long time. As a throat gargle too it has its uses, with a little honey mixed into the infusion or decoction. There is some evidence that if you hold the juice in your mouth for a while it will quieten toothache; the decoction is said to perform the same function.

The herb taken as an infusion or decoction has noticeable benefits for skin tone and tends to clear blemishes from the face. Made into an ointment, the pellitory is very highly thought of as a cure for piles. A poultice of the leaves can be applied with advantage to external injuries of various kinds; and a syrup made from the juice of the herb picked fresh is good for the kidneys. The pollen of the pellitory is one of the first and one of the most active allergens of hay fever and the plant should be avoided by sufferers in early summer — indeed throughout the summer — as the merest touch will cause it to spray the pollen in every direction.

PEPPERMINT —
Mentha piperita
Part used: Leaves

There are many species of mint, all having the same virtues and characteristics, but as the *Mentha piperita* is the one generally used for medicinal purposes, it seems the best species to discuss. A herb which conveys so many obvious blessings was bound to have been noticed in early times. It was very popular with the Romans, who put it in their baths and added it to their wine for the aroma. The women chewed it to conceal the scent of wine on their breaths at a time when women were put to death for partaking of the drink considered fit only for gods and men. Perhaps it should be adopted as the emblem of the Women's Liberation Movement.

Mint has many medicinal benefits, apart from being a universally known remedy for dyspepsia and flatulence — the origin of the after-dinner mint.

Diarrhoea and even cholera respond to the power of mint. In the past it was combined with purgatives to prevent griping. For light colds, mint is the ideal treatment as it will induce perspiration without too much distress. It is frequently used to add an acceptable taste to medicines which would otherwise be unpalatable. An infusion of equal parts of mint, elderflowers and yarrow will remedy influenza within two days without any danger of damaging the heart. Peppermint oil is both anaesthetic and antiseptic and is therefore ideal for the treatment of toothache. Rats are repelled by peppermint and the small flower is an attractive border plant. Plant mint in a container, as it is most invasive. It is also prone to a persistent virus which shows as a 'rust' and will remain in the soil for ever and a day; if your mint begins to rust get rid of it at once.

Herb as food
The herb has a strong flavour. Its leaves are included in salads, jellies and sauces.

For a quick and easy snack see Angelica and mint spread on page 21.

Sparkling mint tea
This makes a pleasant and refreshing drink for children on a hot summer's day. The infu-

sion of the fresh-picked leaves will keep for three or four days in the refrigerator, needing only the addition of lemon juice and soda water to complete the drink. Pick 300 ml (½ pint) of fresh mint leaves, wash them in cold water and put them in a bowl. Pour 1.1 litres (2 pints) of boiling water over the leaves, then cover the bowl and leave to infuse for five minutes. Add two tablespoons of honey and stir until dissolved, then leave to cool. Strain and add the juice of two lemons and sparkling soda water to taste. Do not give chilled drinks to children; see 'Bronchitis', page 109 and also 'Emphysema', page 124.

Mint jelly
Assemble 600 ml (1 pint) of water, 450 g (1 lb) of cooking apples, two cups of freshly picked mint leaves, the juice of one lemon and some sugar. Wash the apples, chop coarsely (do not peel or core), and simmer in the water until the fruit is very soft. Strain the mixture in a jelly-bag overnight. For each 600 ml (1 pint) of juice obtained add 450 g (1 lb) of sugar; put into a saucepan and stir over a gentle heat until the sugar has dissolved, then boil until setting point is reached. Allow to cool and then stir in the lemon juice and the finely chopped mint. Seal in small glass jars.

PLANTAIN, COMMON —
Plantago major
Parts used: Root, leaves, flower-spikes

The plantain is a rather common-looking herb — indeed it would probably be described by many people as a weed — but from time immemorial it has been respected for its healing powers by those 'in the know'. Ancient physicians praised it; Shakespeare makes several references to its powers of healing. It was known in medieval times as a plant of many remedies.

French peasants eat the fresh leaves in salads with dandelion leaves as a kind of inner spring-cleaning. They also apply the juice of the leaves to wounds and cuts. The leaves can be made into very effective poultices for varicose ulcers and other outbreaks of the skin; the juice of the leaves gives ease from insect bites. A decoction is helpful for all ailments of the respiratory tract and for tuberculosis. The plantain was an element in old recipes for ointments. Plantain juice mixed with lemon is an excellent diuretic. The leaves, powdered and taken in water, were thought to eliminate worms. The powdered seed stops vomiting and was once used as a cure for epilepsy, convulsions, jaundice and obstruction of the liver. There are many species of plantain apart from the common plantain and the seeds recommended for the above-mentioned remedies come from the plantain Psyllium or Plantago psyllium. These seeds can often be bought from chemists and sometimes from health food shops. An infusion of plantain, taken internally, is a remedy for piles.

PRIMROSE —
Primula vulgaris
Part used: Root, herb

This most charming of spring flowers also has several medicinal abilities. The whole herb is used when fresh and the root when dried. The roots should be from two- or three-year-old plants and should be thoroughly but rapidly cleaned in cold water, with all small fibres removed. In ancient times the primrose was considered an infallible cure for gout and muscular rheumatism, and a remedy for hysteria. It was taken for those complaints in the form of an infusion made from the petals. Nowadays this infusion is taken for headaches brought on by nerves. The leaves of the primrose were thought an excellent salve for wounds. Rice was often garnished with honey and various herbs, the primrose among them. The entire primrose plant has expectorant qualities and an infusion would help in clearing the lungs and head of catarrh. The family of the primrose gives rise to a quite extraordinary number of hybrids and relations in various directions, from the cowslip to the various garden primulae. One of these is the oxlip, which was once called the *Herba paralysis*, as were its relatives the cowslip and the primrose, because of its reputation for curing several diseases. Thus, for all its innocent loveliness, the primrose packs a punch.

Herb as food
Pickled primroses
This recipe is taken from *The English Housewife* of 1615:

After they have been pickt clean from their stalks and the white ends clean cut away, and washed and dried, And taking a glass pot like a gally-pot, or for want thereof a gally-pot itself And first strew a little crushed white sugar in the bottom Lay a layer of the flower, Then cover that layer over with sugar. Then another layer of flowers and another of sugar. And this do one above the other until the pot do be filled. And ever and

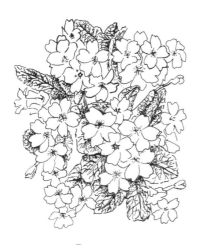

Primrose

anon pressing them hard down with your hand: This done you shall take the best and sharpest vinegar you can get (and if the vinegar be distilled vinegar the flowers will keep their colour the better). And with it fill up your pot till the vinegar swim aloft. Then stop up the pot close, and set in a dry and temperate place.

Serve as a side dish with salad and use at the rate of a teaspoonful for each helping.

RASPBERRY —
Rubus idaeus
Parts used: Leaves, fruit

The raspberry grows freely in Europe. The main difference between the wild and the cultivated variety is one of size, the latter being much the larger. In past times raspberry vinegar was used to ward off the plague; how effectively we cannot be certain. Apart from being a delectable dessert fruit, the raspberry has many virtues. Raspberry syrup makes a marvellous drink for feverish patients. It also, like apple cider vinegar, dissolves the tartar which accumulates on teeth. Raspberry vinegar, an acid syrup made with the juice of the fruit, white wine vinegar and sugar, can be used as a gargle for a sore throat or drunk by feverish patients. Raspberry leaf tea is also effective as a gargle for mouth and throat, and can cleanse ulcers and wounds. The leaves, mixed with powdered slippery elm bark, can be applied as a poultice for burns. An infusion of the leaves is extremely beneficial for chills and influenza, and a decoction of the leaves soothes sore eyes. The raspberry leaf mixed with strawberry, balm, sweet woodruff and bramble leaves and the flowers of the lime tree makes a delicious and effective tea for people who are nervous or suffer from insomnia. Raspberry leaf tea is very valuable during childbirth; it should be taken freely — warm.

If you are planting raspberries, remember that those raised from layers are preferable to those raised from suckers. Plants should be 60 cm (2 feet) apart with 150 cm (5 feet) between rows. Cut out the dead wood in late autumn. Move your raspberries if possible every five years and the quality of the fruit will remain high.

Herb as food
Raspberry jam
An unusual jam is made with 450 g (1 lb) of raspberries, 300 ml (½ pint) of water, 55 g (2 oz) each of chopped nuts and chopped raisins, two sliced oranges and 450 g (1 lb) of sugar. Put all the ingredients into a saucepan and heat gently, stirring constantly, until the sugar has dissolved. Increase the heat to boil the jam but keep stirring until it thickens, then transfer to warmed jam jars and seal.

If raspberries are not too plentiful mix them with other fruits to make jams. Use at the rate of 900 g (2 lbs) of raspberries to 450 g (1 lb) of rhubarb. Combine in a saucepan with 1.1 kg (2½ lbs) of sugar and 600 ml (1 pint) of water. Heat, gently stirring all the time until the sugar is dissolved, then boil to setting point, pot and seal.

ROSE, DOG —
Rosa canina
Part used: Fruit

Neither the leaves nor the flowers of this lovely 'First Rose of Summer' are of much medicinal value, but the fruit more than compensates for this lack.

Rose-hip syrup is a time-honoured means of capturing the vitamin C stored up by the dog rose during the long, sunny days of summer. Many were the expeditions on autumn days long ago to gather the fruit of the dog rose, especially during the world wars, when fruit from faraway sunny lands was not available. The seeds of the rose-hip, dried and powdered, are an ancient remedy for kidney stones and renal colic. Dry the seeds in the sun and infuse. The down or hair which you find on the seeds and which can irritate the skin is a completely safe means of killing the lumbricoid ascaris, a parasite found in the small intestine. Take a pinch coated with honey on an empty stomach. The flesh around the seeds can be dried (not in the sun) and stored until the spring, when it makes a cleansing medicine for the blood. It has a high vitamin C content, cures bleeding gums and provides protection from colds, influenza and the various infections of chest, head and throat which, increasingly, seem to be following us out of the winter and taking longer to shake off in the spring and early summer.

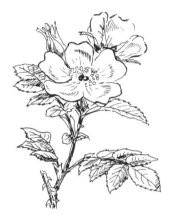

Dog Rose

Herb as food
Rose-hip syrup
Pick the rose-hips and prepare them as quickly as possible in order to preserve the vitamin C. Wash the hips and put them in a saucepan, adding just enough water to cover them. Bring to the boil and simmer until the hips are soft, then, taking the saucepan off the heat, mash them against the side of the pan with the back of a wooden spoon. Strain through a jelly-bag. On the following morning, measure the liquid and for every 600 ml (1 pint) add 225 g (½ lb) of sugar. Heat gently, stirring all the time until the sugar has dissolved, then boil for about five minutes. Skim and pour into clean, warmed bottles with screw-tops. Screw on the caps, leaving them slightly loose, then stand the bottles on a folded cloth (or newspaper) in a deep saucepan. Fill the saucepan with warm water up to the necks of the bottles. Make sure that the bottles do not touch each other. Bring the water to the boil and simmer for ten minutes, then lift the bottles out carefully and tighten the caps. When cold store in a cool, dark place.

To make a summer drink for children add soda water to two tablespoonfuls of the syrup. It also makes a topping for milk puddings or ice cream poured straight from the bottle.

ROSEMARY —
Rosmarinus officinalis
Parts used: Herb, root

Rosemary is an aromatic, shrubby herb with wreaths of small, blue flowers. The emblem of faithfulness in love, it was used in olden times at both weddings and funerals; churches were decorated with rosemary and brides wore rosemary wreaths. Rosemary was a favourite plant in Tudor kitchen gardens, both for decoration and as a pot herb; and it was used to give flavour to wine. It was even burnt as incense, as is evidenced by its old French name, 'Incensier'.

Boiled in wine and inhaled, rosemary was once taken for 'weakness of the brain', whatever that might have been. The flowers had the reputation of preserving clothes from the depredations of the dreaded moth. Sops of rosemary leaves steeped in white wine were prescribed for the restoration of appetite; and the leaves boiled in water and tied around the legs in bandages were supposed to relieve gout. The more serious herbal remedies of today include rosemary as a cure for stomach upsets and headache. It is also used as a hair restorative. The dried plant, leaves and flowers, infused with borax and used cold, is an excellent hairwash, protecting against dandruff. The young tops, both the leaves and flowers, infused and drunk warm, remedy headaches and nervous disorders and also chills and colds. Take care to prevent the steam of the infusion from escaping during preparation as you will otherwise lose the main virtues of the liquid. Rosemary is one of the ingredients in the perfume Eau-de-Cologne.

Herb as food

Rosemary's subtle and elegant flavour enhances a wide range of dishes. Leaves, or even sprigs, inserted into joints of veal or roast lamb or added to chicken stuffing lend an incomparable quality to the finished dish. Chop the leaves and include them in vegetable dishes; they are especially effective with peas, potatoes and marrows. They make a distinctive contribution to the flavour of soups and stews, and go well with fish and rabbit. Put some in a casserole or in a roasting tin and remove before serving. A note of caution: for all its delicacy of flavour, rosemary is rather strong so use a light hand.

Rosemary cheese fingers
In a saucepan melt 55 g (2oz) of butter, then add 170 g (6 oz) of oat-flakes, 170 g (6 oz) of grated Cheddar cheese, one beaten egg and one tablespoonful of finely chopped rosemary. Mix all well together and press into a greased baking tin. Bake in a moderate oven for about half an hour and then cut into fingers.

Oranges with rosemary
Put three or four sprigs of rosemary into a saucepan with 300 ml (½ pint) of water and a half-cup of honey. Heat slowly, stirring all the time, then boil fast for a few minutes and leave to cool. Peel and slice five oranges, arrange them in a dish

and pour the syrup over them. Garnish with a few rosemary flowers.

Rosemary sauce
For a sauce to serve with roast chicken mix the juice of a lemon, a tablespoonful of honey and a tablespoonful of chopped rosemary. Warm the sauce before serving.

Rosemary scones
Take 225 g (½ lb) of self-raising flour, one tablespoonful of butter, one tablespoonful of finely chopped rosemary, a little milk and a tablespoonful of honey. Mix all the dry ingredients in a bowl, then stir in the honey and enough milk to make a soft dough. Roll lightly, cut into scones and bake in a hot oven.

SAGE —
Salvia officinalis
Parts used: Leaves, whole herb

The name of sage comes from '*salvare*', Latin for 'to cure', and sage bids fair to be among the greatest of all the healing herbs. The Romans considered it a sacred herb and surrounded its harvesting with all kinds of ceremonies. They specified that it must not be cut with iron tools, a stricture which might seem odd and unnecessary had we not in recent times discovered that sage is chemically incompatible with iron salts.

Sage was once prescribed for women who had difficulty in conceiving, and there are accounts from ancient sources claiming dramatic restoration of population levels when the sacred herb had been taken. In our time sage retains many of its traditional medicinal uses. An infusion of the dried leaves is a well-known aid to digestion. In warmer countries pork and veal are covered with sage leaves while they are roasting. This makes the meat tastier and easier to digest, and prevents bacterial contamination. A decoction of sage leaves taken fairly hot is a most effective gargle for sore throats. It is also a first-class mouthwash for mouth ulcers, sore gums and dental abscesses. An unguent of sage has good restorative powers when massaged into stiff joints; it alleviates rheumatism, sciatica and tightness of the muscles. Sage has beneficial effects on the blood, liver and stomach. Externally, an infusion can be used as a lotion for ulcers and abrasions. Sage's healing virtues, including its strong antiseptic qualities, would require a book to themselves. No garden should be without it.

Herb as food

Sage has a strong distinctive flavour. Its leaves are excellent in stuffings, particularly for duck, goose and pork. They go well with pea soup, sausages, the pastry for meat pies, and some cheeses.

Sage oatcakes

Put 55 g (2 oz) of butter and six tablespoonfuls of water in a saucepan and heat until the butter has melted. Take it off the heat and mix in 225 g (½ lb) of flake oatmeal, one tablespoonful of chopped sage leaves and a quarter-teaspoonful of bread soda. Mix to a soft dough, adding a little more water if necessary. Place on a greased baking tray and bake for about half an hour, then cut into squares.

Sage and nut pâté

Take 225 g (½ lb) each of ground nuts and cream cheese, one clove of crushed garlic, two tablespoonfuls of olive oil, about four tablespoonfuls of milk and one tablespoonful of chopped sage. Beat all the ingredients together in a bowl, adding enough milk to make a fairly moist mixture. Divide into small bowls and let stand for a while before serving to allow the flavours to combine.

Leek tart with sage

Use 450 g (1 lb) of leeks, one egg, one tablespoonful of chopped parsley, one tablespoonful of chopped sage and three rashers. Line a flan tin with shortcrust pastry. Chop leeks and cook gently in a pan with one tablespoonful of butter, add the herbs, beaten egg and a little milk. Put the mixture into the pastry-lined flan tin and sprinkle the chopped rashers on top. Cook in a medium oven for twenty minutes.

St John's Wort —
Hypericum perforatum
Parts used: Flowers, herb tops

This lovely yellow-flowered plant grows to a height of 45 cm (18 inches) and is found, sometimes in large colonies, along roadsides, in woods and in meadows. If you press the flowers a fragrant red juice will cover your hands; this juice was anciently associated with the blood of Christ. An infusion of the flowers in olive oil produces the very best oil possible for healing wounds. St John's Wort oil keeps its healing properties for two years and is well worth storing as a remedy, not just for open wounds, but for sciatica, lumbago and rheumatism. Back pains of all kinds gain at least some relief from being rubbed with this oil. Children who complain of pains in the stomach are relieved by this oil being rubbed on the affected place. In general the herb has a soothing effect on all ailments of a nervous origin.

Externally, a fomentation of the herb will rid the body of hard tumours and other distortions of the flesh, particularly those resulting from wounds. The oil of St John's Wort has been used with great advantage in healing injured animals as well as people. Very often what cures a human being will also cure an animal — and if not, it won't do it any harm.

SILVERWEED —
Potentilla anserina
Part used: Herb

The silverweed grows by roadsides, in wet pastures and in derelict places. The word *anserina* in its Latin name comes from 'anser' or goose, for geese love this plant; pigs will also seek out its root voraciously. In fact sheep are the only farm animals which will avoid the silverweed. The yellow flower of the herb is particularly lovely in its setting of silver.

All parts of this herb are used medicinally. It should be gathered in June, in dry weather, and dried in half-shade. An infusion of silverweed will stop piles from bleeding and should be drunk at the same time as being applied externally. This infusion, with perhaps a little honey added, makes a gargle for ailments of the throat. Silverweed is used to dispel gravel and a decoction of the herb, taken several times per day, is said to cure jaundice. A decoction is a remedy for mouth ulcers and spongy gums and helps to fix loose teeth in place. It will also act as a lotion for cleaning up the skin. An infusion will ease cramps in the abdomen and heart, especially when accompanied by compresses applied externally to the affected part.

The silverweed has yet more uses; it was anciently and most famously used to stop many forms of inward bleeding. Running sores were dried up and healed by it, and fomentations of the herb were even used to prevent pitting by smallpox. While not an invariable rule, it is often the case that a herb in such demand among the animals of the farm has much to offer man. But again, caution is the watchword. Goats thrive on plants which would instantly kill humans and many other animals.

SORREL —
Rumex acetosa
Parts used: Leaves, herb

Sorrel is a tall-growing herb (about 60 cm/2 feet), found in meadows and most frequently in places where there is iron in the soil. The roots lie very deep in the ground. The leaves of the sorrel are often taken in salad, though be warned that the oxalic acid in the plant can lead to gravel or small stones of calcium oxalate. People with a rheumatic tendency, sufferers from stomach pains, asthma and pulmonary ailments should not take sorrel. Neither, for that matter, should they take certain varieties of spinach which are similarly strong in oxalates.

For those who can take sorrel without fear, it is of great benefit in a wide range of conditions. It is said to sharpen the appetite, to make the heart stronger and to kill worms. Fever and thirst are both allevi-ated by sorrel. A decoction of the herb has long been used in compresses for cuts that won't heal and sores and ulcers of various kinds.

Herb as food
Sorrel has a sharp flavour. Its leaves bring lettuce to life and can be mixed with spinach. Use sparingly. The leaves make a most suitable dressing for roast lamb, and are splendid in soup. In Ireland the sorrel leaves were commonly taken with fish and milk. To rid the sorrel of its acid oxalate and thereby render it edible for people with gout, put the herb into boiling water for three minutes and then throw out the water. If you are making cheese and cannot get rennet, remember that sorrel will curdle milk and can be used instead.

SPHAGNUM MOSS —
Sphagnum cymbifolium
Part used: All

Sphagnum moss was used at no less celebrated an event than the battle of Clontarf in 1014; it is recorded that the wounded on both sides packed moss into their wounds. They did so with good reason, for the sphagnum has a million little tubes and capillaries which make it marvellously absorbent — a capacity which renders it indispensable to our ecology. It absorbs water both from the bogs, high and low, where it grows and from the atmosphere, holding it in its extraordinarily sensitive cells until the moment has come to release it. In this way it plays a considerable role in the regulation of our streams and rivers.

The use of sphagnum moss as a dressing for wounds was rediscovered accidentally by the Germans during the First World War; the Allies were quick to copy them. The dressing was improved by soaking the moss in oil which had been squeezed from garlic and diluted with distilled water; for some reason, this was particularly effective in preventing complications in wounds. One of the ironies of the wartime industry in sphagnum moss was that, in a munitions factory in Scotland, the machine which was used for moulding shells was also used to compress the moss into cakes for convenience in transporting it to the trenches on mainland Europe.

STRAWBERRY —
Fragaria vesca
Part used: Leaves

The strawberry, either wild or cultivated, is a pendent plant that likes to grow half in and half out of shade. Its natural habitat is a south-facing bank on the edge of woodlands. The notion that its name comes from the practice of putting straw beneath the berries to protect them from the earth is mistaken. The 'straw' is really 'strew', which is what the plant does with its mat of vines.

Strawberries and cream are a welcome part of our diet in early summer, viewed as a luxury bestowed by nature to celebrate the coming of long, sunny days. But there is much more to the strawberry than this. The fruit is good for people in feverish conditions. It has properties which tend to dissolve gall and kidney stones. Strawberries relieve both constipation and gastro-enteritis; their seeds have a stimulating effect on bowel action. An infusion of the leaves stops dysentery. The fresh strawberry will remove discoloration from teeth: leave the juice on the teeth for five to ten minutes, then clean with warm water and a brush dipped in bicarbonate of soda. A decoction of the root is a remedy for dysentery, diarrhoea, cystitis, jaundice, bronchitis and arthritis. Strawberries are a time-honoured beauty treatment. Rub the face with strawberries before going to bed and remove the juice in the morning with clean warm water. Constant handling of strawberries — even strawberry poultices on the hands — in summer is said to prevent chilblains in the winter.

SUMMER SAVORY —
Satureia hortensis
Part used: Herb

This hardy herb is among the most fragrant of all plants and is sometimes grown near bee-hives in the hope that it will impart its aroma to the honey. It is raised from seeds which are sown in April. Used in past centuries in the making of conserves and syrups, it is yet another of the pot herbs which have medicinal as well as culinary virtues. Imparting flavour to pork pies and sausages, green peas and many other delights of the kitchen, summer savory provides an alternative to chervil and parsley when these are not available.

Summer savory is sometimes combined with medicines, to which it lends warmth and fragrance. Sufferers from colic and flatulence are known to benefit from summer savory, and the juice of the herb is good for eyes and ears. The removal of catarrh from the chest and lungs is another of its virtues. Summer savory is recommended as bringing relief to wasp and bee stings, but as in the case of the marigold, this may be questionable. The ancient Romans used vinegar flavoured with summer savory in the circumstances in which we use mint sauce. There is no harm in trying the summer savory, even in combination with other herbs, to flavour your vinegar, but always remember that in culinary as in medicinal matters, a little of a herb goes a long way. Herbs are concentrations, generally the opposites and complementaries of the foods which we eat in large amounts, adding quality to the quantity. There are of course, some herbs, like comfrey and fennel, which are taken in bulk as vegetables.

Herb as food
Be sure to distinguish between summer savory and winter savory when it comes to flavouring food, for while they both have a peppery taste the winter savory is much stronger and must be used with restraint. The sprigs of summer savory may be boiled with broad beans and green beans, and the

chopped leaves can be included in a sauce for fish and tomatoes. They can also be added to stews and used to flavour pork and veal chops. They are said to go well with poultry and can be included in salads.

TANSY —
Tanacetum vulgare
Part used: Leaves, herb

This herb reaches 60 or even 90 cm (2–3 feet) in height and stands very erect. It has flat yellow flowers and long leaves. Tansy will grow in almost any part of any garden. Tansy cakes were made in olden times at Easter when the flowers were fresh and new; they were thought to restore the body after the Lenten fasting. A great deal of salt fish was taken in Lent in those days and tansy was believed necessary to normalise the system after this fairly stern fare. Tansy tea was sometimes taken during Lent for the same purpose. The main, but by no means only, medicinal use of tansy is as a vermifuge for children. An infusion should be taken in teacupful doses fasting, morning and night. The fresh leaves of the herb, pounded and applied as a poultice externally, can sometimes suffice to expel the worms. A poultice of tansy can

be used for some skin problems and will benefit sprains and swellings. An infusion applied hot as a fomentation will relieve rheumatism. Tansy has also been used to heal wounds. Tansy leaves, fresh or dried, are sometimes put between sheet and mattress to keep beds free of bugs and fleas. The same can be done with kennels to keep the straw clear of unwelcome visitors. Tansy is a herb of great power and efficacy. In large and very strong doses it can be a severe irritant and can cause vertigo and cramps. However, a little thought and common sense should easily prevent such discomfort.

TARRAGON —
Artemisia dracunculus
Parts used: Leaves, herb

The name is derived from the Latin for 'Little dragon' and, like all herbs which have the word 'dragon' in their names, it was believed to contain the antidote to all manner of venomous bites and stings. Tarragon favours a rather poor, dry soil and in these more northerly regions it generally requires heat to get over the winter.

Tarragon is a pot herb with some medicinal uses. It is good for nausea, bad digestion and flatulence, and will ease rheumatic pain. At one time the root of tarragon was used to cure toothache.

Herb as food

People on a salt-free diet find tarragon has a stimulating effect on their digestive systems without causing them any irritation. A more common use for it in some Eastern countries is as an appetiser. In France cooks always mix mustard with tarragon vinegar. To make this, pick the leaves on a dry day shortly before the herb flowers. Dry the leaves briefly and then put them in a jar, cover them with vinegar and let nature take its course for a few hours. Then strain the mix through a jelly-bag and seal in bottles. For the best result use the best white vinegar you can get.

The Moors who conquered Spain brought this liquorice-tasting herb into Europe. Like most North Africans they were experts in seasoning. Try a little on the Sunday joint or sprinkled on salads. Tarragon butter (made like garlic butter) goes very well with shellfish, mushrooms, artichokes, tomatoes, courgettes, broccoli and beetroot, and is also said to complement cold egg dishes. Tarragon is used in sauces for fish and is an ingredient of fines herbes, a mixture of some of the more distinguished cooking herbs, which are dried, mixed and kept in the kitchen to be added to various dishes.

THYME —
Thymus vulgaris
Part used: Herb

Garden thyme comes in several varieties and is universally popular as a pot herb. Bees love it. In the Middle Ages thyme symbolised action and courage; ladies embroidered scarves with a bee working a sprig of thyme and presented them to their knightly lovers as a spur to performing gallant deeds. Thyme was used to add flavour to cheese by the Romans.

Thyme is yet another popular pot herb which also confers medicinal benefits. Pound the herb and add anything from 30 to 170 g (1 to 6 oz) to a syrup and you have a cure for whooping cough. An infusion of the herb will achieve the same result taken in tablespoonfuls several times a day. Complaints which are alleviated by thyme include insomnia, urinary tract infections, asthma, bronchitis, influenza, bad digestion, distension, cardiac weakness, anaemia and general exhaustion of the system. The decoction is a good hair lotion and is reputed to prevent baldness. Infusion of thyme is a remedy for wind in the stomach. It is also useful in feverish conditions. An ointment of the herb is said to remove warts and swellings of various kinds. Thyme is a very safe herb, taken in sensible amounts. In herbal medicines, it is generally used in combination with other remedies, but even on its own it has a wide range of applications. Keep thyme roots well protected in winter by earthing them up.

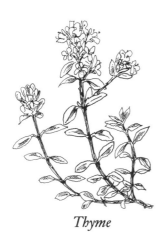

Thyme

Herb as food
Common thyme is strongly if pleasantly flavoured. Lemon thyme is lighter and, as its name implies, has a lemon flavour. Thyme leaves are used to advantage in stuffings and with rabbit, turkey, chicken and veal. Salads benefit from a light shake of thyme. Among the vegetables, it enhances the flavour of aubergines, onions, carrots, beetroots and tomatoes. Thyme is also sometimes taken with fish.

TOADFLAX —
Linaria vulgaris
Part used: Herb

This wild and slightly dishevelled member of the long-tailed and distinguished family of the Linaria takes its name from the toad, to which its flowers are said to bear some resemblance. The combination of orange and yellow in its flowers have given it the nickname 'Eggs and Bacon'. It has long been a medicinal herb.

Toadflax taken as an infusion has very strong purgative effects, and in cases of jaundice, liver and skin diseases, it has proved a most powerful remedy. But be warned: the infusion is a fairly awful-tasting brew. A decoction of the leaves and flowers will serve the same purpose, the addition of a little cinnamon and quinine rendering it more effective. The juice of the toadflax was once commonly used for washing ulcers and an ointment made from the herb is beneficial for skin complaints and piles. A poultice is also sometimes applied to piles.

Toadflax can be grown easily, though as with many herbs, it is so healthy that it must be controlled; otherwise it will take over and be called a weed. Most of what are termed weeds have many uses, cosmetic, culinary and medicinal. Perhaps a little less obsession with clean-shaven lawns and a little more indulgence towards what we insist on calling weeds would add some interest to our gardens — say a corner with a few nettles, dandelions, docks, and anything else that might meander in from the great wilderness beyond.

VALERIAN —
Valeriana officinalis
Part used: Root

There are approximately 150 species of valerian but when spoken of medicinally it is the *Valeriana officinalis* that is meant. Called 'All Heal' in the Middle Ages because of its curative powers, the valerian has tall stems and unmistakable pink, or sometimes white, flowers and grows in wet places near rivers and ditches. The flowers bloom from June to September.

Valerian, only the root of which is used medicinally, is very effectively employed as a sedative in cases of nervous upset, St Vitus's dance and nerve pains of various kinds.

People who suffer from nervous overstrain are especially well served by the herb as it has none of the undesirable after-effects of narcotics; however, large doses can induce headache. Valerian is often given as a tincture. It is used as a sedative for nervous ailments, including vapours, vertigo, palpitations, nervous contractions of the stomach and insomnia. It is also given to children with convulsions, as a powder taken with honey. Weakened eyesight is said to benefit from valerian.

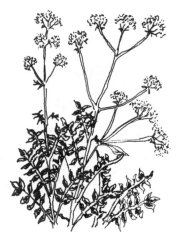

Valerian

In 1592 one Fabius Calumna is reported as having healed himself of epilepsy by taking this very versatile herb. According to an ancient recipe, valerian root, boiled with liquorice, raisins and aniseed, is good for a persistent cough. The root has also been used as a spice, a perfume and a pot herb. It was a particularly popular addition to broths and stews in the border country between England and Scotland in former centuries.

VERVAIN —
Verbena officinalis
Parts used: Leaves, flowering heads

Whether in pagan or in Christian times, vervain has ever been the herb most closely associated with magic and mystique. The Romans credited it with being able to revive the fires of love and consequently called it the 'luck of Venus'. The druids in early Celtic times cleansed their altars with vervain before offering sacrifice. It was used to prophesy, to protect against evil spirits and to accompany various spells and incantations.

The leaves and flowering heads of the vervain are employed medicinally. The instincts of the ancients prove as accurate as ever; the herb is used in healing over thirty ailments. Internally the vervain is taken as a decoction. It is recommended for fever, gravel, flatulence, jaundice and ailments of the kidney, and also said to be of help with pleurisy and ulcers. Externally, as a poultice, it has benefited people with rheumatism, ear-neuralgia and headache; sometimes it is applied externally for piles. The decoction is also used in compresses for wounds and ulcers, as a mouthwash for inflamed gums and as a gargle for sore throats. A poultice of vervain plant has been applied with success to lumbago. Extraordinary results have been achieved by the use of vervain in the treatment of tumours of a certain kind, but further work is necessary before any claims can be made on this account. A decoction of vervain taken in a day is said to be a successful purge, but purging is an affair to be approached with care and under medical supervision. In general, the gentler the cure for any condition, the more natural and therefore the better.

WALNUT —
Juglans nigra
Parts used: Leaves, bark

The walnut comes originally from Persia, Juglans meaning 'Jupiter's nuts', for Jupiter was said to have lived on walnuts in the Golden Age when men lived on acorns — so much more highly than the oak was the walnut valued in early times. The delicious nut needs no introduction but it is equalled in medicinal efficacy by the leaves and bark, which are used in the treatment of skin ailments. Eczema and herpes are healed by two or three cupfuls of decoction of the leaves drunk between meals. Other complaints said to be remedied by this decoction are pulmonary conditions, rheumatism, anaemia, and disorders of the digestive tract such as gastroenteritis. Night sweats and diabetes are also thought to benefit. Externally the decoction is added to footbaths and handbaths for chilblains and excessive perspiration, and used as a lotion for skin problems, varicose ulcers and problems of the eyes, e.g. styes, irritation of the eyelids and ophthalmia.

The leaves of the walnut have an extremely strong smell which can cause discomfort to those highly sensitive to such things, even though the smell is quite pleasant. An old cure for a stubborn varicose ulcer is to apply sugar which has been soaked in a decoction of walnut leaves. The bark of the walnut, dried and powdered, is an effective purgative when taken in an infusion. The juice of the green husks of the nuts boiled with honey makes a wholesome gargle for sore mouths or throats. The leaves should be picked carefully before the middle of July and dried in shade, then packed in airtight containers.

WOOD SANICLE —
Sanicula europaea
Part used: Herb

The wood sanicle is closely related to the common bugle. It grows up to 60 cm (2 feet) tall and has tiny pink-white flowers. The name 'sanicle' comes from the Latin *'sano'*, meaning 'I heal'. The fame of the sanicle in early times rested on its capacity for healing wounds.

The sanicle is generally combined with other herbs for blood disorders. It is thought to benefit sufferers from diarrhoea and dysentery, and in France is widely used for serious bleeding from the lungs and other organs. It makes a gargle for sore throats and quinsy. Sanicle is most often taken as an infusion, which can also be applied externally. It is very effective when, either as a decoction or as an infusion, it is applied externally to children who are suffering from any kind of rash. It is also most beneficial in lung ailments, serious and prolonged catarrhal infections, diseases of the bronchii — in fact, in all complaints of the chest.

Sanicle acts as a purifier of the blood and thereby speeds up the healing process, whether applied externally or internally. A decoction of the leaves was at one time recommended for bleeding piles; the leaves and roots can be made into an ointment for the relief of this complaint. A compress made from a decoction of the roots will greatly soothe chilblains and general inflammations. The wood sanicle is resorted to less than it once was and deserves to come back into fashion.

YARROW —
Achillea millefolium
Parts used: Whole herb

Achilles at Troy used the yarrow to heal the wounds of his comrades in arms. From this power the yarrow got at least two of its nicknames, Soldiers' Wound Wort and Knights' Milfoil. In Scotland an ointment for wounds is still made from yarrow. In the Orkney Islands yarrow tea is used to chase away the 'blues', presumably when supplies of stronger stuff run out. The French call it the 'herb charpentier' or the carpenter's herb from its ability to draw splinters of wood from the hands.

The yarrow is credited both with stanching a bleeding nose and with making the nose bleed and thereby bringing relief to an aching head. How it can do both is not clear, but the agreed method is simply to roll up a leaf and stuff it in the nostril. For general medicinal purposes the whole plant, stems, leaves and flowers, is used. Yarrow tea is a favourite remedy for severe colds. It encourages perspiration where desired. It may be drunk warm with whatever additives seem appropriate, such as honey, cayenne pepper or even something stronger. A decoction of the whole plant is recommended for disorders of the kidneys and for bleeding piles. Yarrow tea will help to stop bleeding after the extraction of a tooth and in fact is used to stop all internal bleeding. Whether you apply it as a poultice, compress or lotion, yarrow has a marvellous healing effect upon wounds. A decoction of yarrow has the reputation of preventing baldness, though cynics still insist that the only thing that stops falling hair is the floor. Yarrow stimulates the action of the bone marrow in the making of blood.

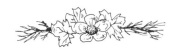

Part II
Ailments

ACNE

Acne is a skin disorder which usually afflicts adolescents. It consists of outbreaks of pimples, the result of sebaceous glands becoming blocked and inflamed. Kidney trouble, nervous tension and various glandular changes associated with puberty all play a part in bringing on these unsightly eruptions. Just as there are many contributory causes, so there are many remedial steps which can be taken. Vitamins A, B complex and E are essential for clear, healthy skin, and zinc has been found very beneficial in some cases. There is also a range of herbal preparations which can assist in a speedy improvement of the condition. Burdock root and dandelion root are two of these. Teenagers often drink a lot of coffee; a switch to dandelion coffee might be of advantage. Camomile tea and limeblossom tea have a calming effect on the nervous system, and, with dandelion coffee, can be purchased in most health food shops. A cream made from the marigold flower is beneficial for greasy skin. Comfrey tea, also available at health food shops, has a healing effect when applied to the skin as a lotion. Soap should be carefully chosen or even avoided. The tea of the stinging nettle has a very cleansing effect on the blood and can be taken several times a day but not over long periods of time (see 'Common Stinging Nettle' on page 71).

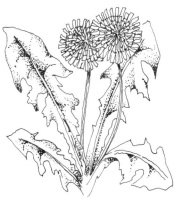

Dandelion

There is an old remedy, for external application, which may be worth a try. Place shredded horseradish in a bottle of wine, leave for some time in temperate conditions. The resulting horseradish vinegar administered to the skin of the face can be of some benefit. The wine becoming vinegar neutralises the heat of the horseradish and the horseradish takes the bitterness out of the vinegar. A decoction of the walnut leaf also makes a good lotion for acne.

Diet plays an important part in healing acne. When possible, vegetables should be eaten raw. It is known that parsley and watercress can have a most beneficial influence. Be careful with the watercress; it frequently grows in the same waters as fool's cress, which, as its name implies, is toxic and should not be eaten. Tender dandelion leaves are also helpful. Plenty of fresh fruit should be eaten and the usual 'suspects' — fried food, white flour, white sugar and its by-products, and chocolate of all kinds — should be sacrified to the greater good. When the pimples have gone but left unsightly scars, break a wheat-germ oil capsule into the cavities; this will significantly assist the healing action.

Before applying a lotion or cream to the face it is necessary to remove the surface oil which blocks the pores and causes the pimples typical of acne. The most effective method is to shake about a teaspoonful of talcum powder (ideally baby talcum powder) into the palm of your hand, add enough warm water to make a soft paste, spread this all over the pimples and allow to dry for a few minutes. The powder will begin to flake off your face. At this stage use a tissue that has been well wetted in lukewarm water to wash off the powder; it will have removed the excess oil from your skin. This paste is very mild and can be applied as often as you like — every day or even twice a day; it is preferable to other types of face pack which would be too astringent to use so often.

After the talcum paste, apply one of the herbal lotions and then a healing cream, such as one made from marigold flower or comfrey.

An old East European tonic for the blood comprises equal parts of lavender, white clover, the petals of the marigold and the soft inner bark of either the beech tree or the elder. Infuse and drink a cupful first thing in the morning; this is thought to clear up acne.

ANAEMIA

Anaemia means that either the number of red blood

cells or the red pigment which carries iron in the blood is below the level required by a healthy bloodstream. The red blood cells ferry oxygen from your lungs to every area of your body. The oxygen combines with iron to make haemoglobin. A lack of oxygen or iron leads to the classic symptoms of anaemia: a faster heartbeat, headaches, general debility. There can be many causes for this condition, including haemorrhage, failure of bone marrow to make new cells, failure of the body to absorb iron in sufficient amounts from food. It can even be a side-effect of drugs being taken for some other complaint. Obviously, anaemia is a matter to be discussed with your medical adviser, but a few ways of improving the condition can be mentioned without trespassing on professional territory.

Firstly, there is the matter of diet. If your diet consists mainly of refined foods, you are not receiving the required amount of iron. There is a further problem when, in a fit of conscience, the manufacturers of these refined foods decide to add iron to their products, for if this is inorganic iron it poses a positive threat to your health. The so-called 'enrichment' and 'fortification' of food with inorganic iron can lead to disable-

ment and even death, according to some medical authorities.

There are several natural foods and herbs that assist in overcoming anaemia. Garlic can kill intestinal parasites, which are far more common than is generally appreciated and which can seriously deplete your blood supplies. Foods which should be taken in as large quantities as is feasible include green leafy vegetables, onions, whole grains and brown rice. Sunflower seeds and lentils, Brazil nuts and almonds are recommended too. Soya beans are a primary source of iron and other minerals. Stinging nettle tea also contains iron and has a cleansing and stimulating effect on the bloodstream. Herbs which contain iron include parsley and alfalfa, watercress and chickweed. (Don't confuse the watercress with fool's cress.) Apples, pears, prunes, raisins and grapes are all beneficial. Strawberry leaf tea, because of its iron content, has a long tradition of use in treating anaemia. Liver produces more iron than any other known food source and blackstrap molasses is a marvellous source of organic iron, with fifteen times as much iron as ordinary molasses. Sweeten it with a little honey and take it with hot water or warm milk going to bed; it will make you sleep and rebuild your blood while you rest. Use warmed rather than boiling milk as boiling milk will curdle when molasses is added.

Beef tea was in former times recommended for anaemia. Cut 450 g (1 lb) of shin beef into cubes and cover with cold water. Leave overnight, then boil and strain. Beef tea is also given to convalescents.

ARTERIOSCLEROSIS

The dreaded cholesterol deposits harden and thicken the artery walls, and if this process continues beyond a critical point, it leads to coronary thrombosis. You should do everything you can to avoid developing this potentially fatal condition. Some people inherit the problem but others bring it upon themselves through eating the wrong foods or through smoking. Fast foods, an excess of animal fat, insufficient consumption of whole grains, salads, vegetables and fresh fruit — all these dietary mistakes contribute to hardening of the arteries.

Fortunately nature supplies us with ample antidotes to the condition. The most efficacious is garlic, which assists in keeping cholesterol levels normal and in reducing deposits of fat inside the blood vessels. It has a cleansing effect on the entire system. Remember you can take garlic in perles or capsules before going to bed and be fit to join the bus queue in the morning. Two perles is the usual dose.

Further help is available in the form of hawthorn, taken as a tea or as a decoction. Infuse the dried flowers, one teaspoonful to a cup of boiling water. This will, over the course of time, bring high blood pressure down to normal as well as acting altogether beneficially on the blood vessels. An alternative method would be to chop the leaves of the hawthorn finely and mix them half and half with ordinary Indian tea. In southern England the leaf of the hop is similarly mixed with tea and has long been popular as a means of controlling blood pressure. Limeblossom tea is sedative and helps to reduce pressure in the arteries by thinning the blood. An infusion of chopped stinging nettles, leaves and stalks, has a most invigorating effect on the entire system as well as being of particular benefit to the arteries. The stinging nettles picked in May are the best ones for drying and storing; in June they will have grown acidic and disagreeable. The dried nettles must remain green or they forfeit their medicinal qualities. Nettle tea is available all the year round from health food and chemists' shops.

The speedwell (*Veronica officinalis*), taken as an infusion, is reputedly remarkable at removing cholesterol from the arteries. Equal parts of marjoram, sage and mint in infusion have been known to bring relief.

If the disease is at an advanced stage it can often be relieved by bathing hands and feet twice daily, in a mixture of two crushed cloves of garlic and handfuls of broom flowers, the leaves of the lesser celandine and the flowers of the hawthorn. Make them up in a decoction and allow them to cool to a comfortable temperature.

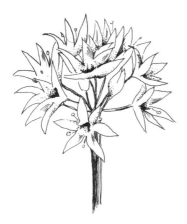

Ramsons (Wild Garlic)

ARTHRITIS

'Arthritis' is thought by many in the medical world to be a heading under which several diseases are collected, and — to complicate matters further — it is widely acknowledged that no two cases of any of these individual diseases are the same. Many reputable medical sources go so far as to say that there is no cure for arthritis. Some who have studied the subject, however, beg to differ.

'Let your medicine be your food and your food your medicine,' wrote Hippocrates, the father of medicine, more than two thousand years ago, and diet is one means of at least alleviating arthritis. Physical and emotional stress, wrong feeding, obesity, calcium deficiency and insufficient hydrochloric acid in the system have been listed as some of the causes of osteo-arthritis, a common and painful form of the disease. According to Dr D.C. Jarvis, who made an extremely instructive study of folk medicine in Vermont, arthritis sufferers are usually said to be calcium-deficient while at the same time accumulating calcium deposits on joints. In Vermont this problem was traced, not to the most obvious source — shortage of calcium in the system — but rather to a shortage of hydrochloric acid in the stomach upon which the proper metabolism of calcium depends. The conclusion would seem to be that the sufferer may well have enough calcium in the system but it simply accumulates in the wrong, and most pain-inducing, places.

Two teaspoons of apple cider vinegar and two of honey in a glass of water taken with each meal is the antidote to the uneven distribution of calcium. You can buy this mixture as Honegar in health food shops.

Remarkable cures have been claimed by practitioners who have moved their patients onto a diet of raw food, i.e. one with no refined, cooked or preserved foods. If you think this might be the answer to your problems, see *A Doctor's Proven New Home Cure for Arthritis* by Dr Giraud Campbell, which gives details of an approach claimed to cure arthritis in seven days.

Several herbs have been found useful in the treatment of arthritis. Ash and comfrey, and especially nettles, taken as infusions, are thought to help; take them all, particularly the nettles, in moderation. An Indian herbal remedy called chaparral, which can be found in health food shops, is said to benefit osteo-arthritis if two tablets are taken each day.

Citrus fruits should be avoided.

An infusion of either meadowsweet or willow bark, taken internally, eases the pains and aches of arthritis. A soothing oil, made by adding one teaspoon of either Olbas oil or rosemary oil to half a cup of sunflower oil, can be massaged into the affected parts.

Pecan nuts, brewer's yeast, bananas and wheatgerm are said to combine well, taken over a period of time, to bring great relief. These ingredients should be readily available; the pecan nuts, wheatgerm and brewer's yeast are usually stocked by health food shops. Considering the pain involved in most arthritic conditions, this recipe is certainly worth a try. Take the various ingredients in small amounts to begin with — say six pecan nuts to a teaspoonful of wheatgerm, a teaspoonful of brewer's yeast and one banana. The mixture could become part of an appetising breakfast muesli.

ASTHMA

Throughout the world there is an alarming multiplication in the incidences of respiratory diseases, including asthma. This is undoubtedly related to the dramatic rise in air pollution which has accompanied industrial development. But these diseases have many and mysterious origins, none more so than asthma. Emotional disturbances and allergies are thought to be among the culprits. So are atmospheric pressure and, possibly, other climatic factors. Even the drug aspirin, provided for our benefit by the meadowsweet, has been found to trigger asthmatic attacks in some sufferers who are, apparently, over-sensitive to it.

One school of medical opinion blames asthma on nutritional deficiency and recommends the consumption of natural fish liver oil because it contains vitamins A and D, of which the sufferers show some shortage. Bone meal, in liberal amounts, is given with these vitamins and the general effect is said to be beneficial to many. But the complex question of vitamins is obviously related to your particular diet, and your practitioner should be able to tell you whether or not the food you are eating can supply your specific requirements. Tissue salts are purportedly another source of relief from asthma, with one known as *Kali. Mur.* said to be of assistance in most cases. These salts are available without prescription in health food and chemists' shops. They are well worth a try and are quite harmless to take.

Of the many herbs which aid in clearing mucus from the asthmatic's head and chest, the volatile oils of eucalyptus, peppermint, cajeput, juniper, wintergreen and clove oils with menthol are combined in a non-drug inhalant, available commercially. A few drops of this combination in a vaporiser relieve the breathing and disinfect the respiratory tract. As a general rule the asthmatic should take garlic in as many ways as possible and also add some comfrey to the diet. Both of these herbs have a long history of benefiting chest and lung complaints. The garlic has a marvellous natural disinfecting quality, and the comfrey promotes healing whether used externally or internally.

Some sufferers from asthma have found that a bedtime hot bath containing pine buds or catmint promotes a restful night's sleep. A vigorous drying with a rough towel after the bath stimulates the skin to perform its function of expelling toxins, thereby taking some strain off the respiratory tract.

Carrageen moss which grows on rocks around the seashore is an age-old remedy for complaints of the respiratory organs, including asthma. The best ways to take this cure are as follows:

Carrageen drink

Put 7 g (¼ oz) of carrageen and the rind and juice of one lemon in 600 ml (1 pint) of water. Bring to the boil and simmer while stirring for about twenty minutes. Strain. Add honey to taste. Serve hot or cold.

Carrageen blancmange

Add 30 g (1 oz) of carrageen and the rind of one lemon to 600 ml (1 pint) of milk and bring to the boil. Simmer for about fifteen minutes, stirring continuously. Strain. Add honey to taste and pour into a wet mould; leave until set. Turn out, decorate and serve.

As a supplement to everyday diet carrageen moss is a most valuable source of the vitamins, minerals and trace elements which have been refined out of processed foods. The blancmange recipe above may provide a convenient way of introducing children to the marvels of carrageen, not least of which will be to protect them from coughs and colds. See also the recipe for carrageen jelly in 'Bronchitis' on page 110.

Another folk cure for asthma is made up by immersing several slices of raw onion in a jar of liquid honey, sealing the jar and allowing it to stand overnight. Take teaspoonfuls of the resultant syrup several times per day. Do not use honey that has crystallised and been heated to liquefy it, as this process will have destroyed the vitamins.

It was once a custom in country houses to sprinkle cold (Indian) tea on the floor before sweeping — for the purpose, it was said, of keeping down the dust. Scientists have recently discovered that the instinct behind this custom was uncannily accurate. The faeces of the house dust mite, invisibly present in every house, provoke asthmatic reactions in the lungs of some people who are particularly sensitive to them. These harmful effects are neutralised by the faeces being sprayed with tannin, which is exactly what was being done by the tea-sprinkling housewives of long ago, for tea contains tannin. Fill a spray-bottle with the cold tea left in your teapot and spray the house with a very fine mist so as not to stain any of the soft furnishings. Do this each time before you use the vacuum cleaner or sweeping brush. Proprietary sprays can be purchased but their active ingredient is tannin which the tea supplies.

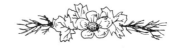

BACKACHE

There are almost as many causes of backache as there are sufferers from backaches — or so it sometimes seems. In reality the main causes of the complaint are often nothing more than lack of exercise and inappropriate diet. However, if symptoms persist, a full medical diagnosis should be sought without delay as they may originate in a disease of some vital organ. Ours is an automated, transported and sedentary society where wheels have almost taken the place of legs and where physical work is largely a matter of pressing buttons. Never was it more vital for a generation to attend to bodily posture and never was less heed paid to this essential aid to good health. Much is written about chairs that do not support us or that catch our bodies at the wrong point. Our grandparents didn't worry about the backs of their chairs — their own backs never touched them at all, so upright did they remain even when seated. High heels force the body forward and put the spine out of alignment. Inexperienced lifting throws weight on the spine that should be carried by the legs. Golf, which is the standard form of relaxation for the walking wounded of commerce, too often causes the kind of stress that leads to backache.

An excess of carbohydrate foods tends to make muscles flabby. A proper diet, coupled with a few very straightforward exercises to strengthen the muscles of the abdomen, has been known to cure more backaches than you might imagine. It helps if you don't always sit on the same chair. Driving long distances without a break can induce back pain. Even something as simple as poring over a book when you should probably have your eyes tested for reading glasses can put stress on your neck, which in turn affects the back.

There are complaints of the back which are serious and will not be cured by either proper diet or exercise, but these are rare. The main problems are caused by postural and alignment faults, and you can benefit greatly from seeing an osteopath or a chiropractor (who can sometimes rectify a backache within minutes). Common sense plays a major part in helping you to understand and correct your backache. While your doctor can describe the mechanics of the spine and explain the problem, only you can take the appropriate action — meaning exercise — to put matters right.

Spasmodic back pains are sometimes remedied by taking magnesium phosphate, a biochemic tissue salt. This is available without prescription from chemists' and health food shops under the name of Mag. Phos. and is very safe to use. Tissue salts in general bear investigation; look out for books on Dr Scheussler's biochemic cures.

Do not underestimate the therapeutic value of warmth and rest in the treatment of backache. Several patent liniments can be bought from chemists' or health food shops.

A herbal remedy that has for many a day brought relief to strained muscles is made up by gently heating St John's Wort which has been covered with olive oil for fifteen minutes in a steel pan. Strain the oil when it cools, and massage gently into the affected part. This may be available already made up in health food shops, where you will probably find a collection of such oils.

An infusion of yarrow, drunk fairly hot, has the reputation of easing rheumatic pain in the back. Do not allow back pain to persist for too long without seeing a doctor.

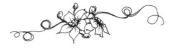

Blood Disorders

The blood becomes impure and sluggish over the winter months, particularly in our climate, and needs a spring-cleaning. Nettle tea and nettles eaten as a vegetable are among nature's great cleansers of the blood. A decoction of red clover flowers, clivers, fumitory, burdock root, dandelion root and bogbean, taken internally, will significantly improve the blood; celery and watercress also have a salutary effect. But there are many herbs which help to purify the bloodstream, each working from a slightly different angle. They combine to provide a thoroughly cleansed and vigorous blood supply so you can enjoy the delights of summer and autumn before facing the rigours of another winter.

The common plantain (*Plantago major*), which should be taken as an infusion, is said to cleanse the blood better than any other herb. It also cleanses the stomach and lungs, and because, in the complex interactions of the body, all these processes are connected, many related purposes are served by the one herb. An infusion of the petals of the cowslip flower has the particular virtue of ridding the blood of those toxic substances which lead to the conditions of gout and rheumatism in its various forms. Ramsons, or wild garlic, remove those toxins which are related to herpes, eczema and scrofula. The leaves can be used in stews or even in sandwiches. A surprisingly tasty drink can be made by boiling finely chopped leaves in 250 ml (9 fl oz) of white wine. Restore the sweetness of the wine with honey and sip slowly. The speedwell can be added to any blood-cleansing tea. The leaves of the walnut (*Juglans nigra*) taken as a tea will cleanse the blood and tend to rectify intestinal disorders. The yarrow (*Achillea millefolium*) has a strong effect on the marrow of the bones, stimulating the renewal of the blood; it too should be taken as a tea. Nature provides a broad range of blood-cleansing herbs in the spring, just when we need them most.

Blood poisoning requires immediate professional attention, but all the above remedies will help to prevent a return of the malady.

The flowers of marigold taken as an infusion both cleanse the blood and stimulate the circulation. An infusion of sage will also purify the blood.

Pick the flower shoots of the elder while they are still green and unopened, mix one tablespoonful of the elder with one tablespoonful of cowslip flower and a teaspoonful each of stinging nettle and dandelion root. Infuse one heaped teaspoonful of the mixture in a mug of boiling water for three minutes. Strain and drink. Take a mug of this mixture every day for ten days as a spring blood tonic. For information on digging dandelion roots see 'Dandelion' on page 41-2.

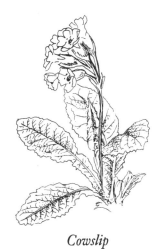

Cowslip

BLOOD PRESSURE

If you think you have a problem with your blood pressure consult a medical practitioner. Normal blood pressure, like health itself, is a state of equilibrium between extremes. The more troublesome and more common extreme is high blood pressure, which has a variety of causes — hardened arteries, heart disease, psychological difficulties or dietary mistakes of one kind or another. In this latter connection, bear in mind that ordinary tea, or so-called Indian tea, when taken in its 'strong' form, and even when taken excessively in its weaker forms, is most detrimental to the blood pressure. It causes a sudden raising of the pressure followed by a sharp fall as the effects wear off. This, any doctor will tell you, is a matter to be taken very seriously. A half-and-half admixture of finely chopped hawthorn leaves or hop leaves will offset or neutralise this effect. Garlic will lower both the blood pressure and the cholesterol level of the blood. Stinging nettle and yarrow are thought to be effective against the rise in blood pressure brought on by stress. The modern world is a very stressful place. The words 'adrenalin' and 'manic' have entered our everyday vocabulary, along with several other stress-related terms. Popular entertainment, including sport, grows more violent with each year that passes; and competition has become a value in itself and not merely a by-product of healthy thinking. This permanent and universal disturbance of the tranquillity to which we

all aspire can only have the effect of driving up blood pressure; a return to religious and philosophical ideas of our destiny might not be the least effective cure. Animal fats, alcohol, coffee and tea will have to go if blood pressure is to be lowered. Recommended foods are raw salads, fresh fruit and green leafy vegetables — in other words, those which seem to be good for everything.

Low blood pressure is often perfectly normal unless it first occurs after an illness. Of the many herbs that help to raise it, ginseng is said to be among the most effective.

An infused mixture of the following herbs in equal parts will assist in regulating the blood pressure: basil, camomile, mint and vervain. Sip a cupful at night before going to bed.

Keep a pot of chives growing on your windowsill and use the chopped leaves or 'grass' as a flavouring; they are especially tasty in omelettes, sandwiches and soup. Mildly antibiotic and a stimulant for the appetite, the leaves are a painless means of helping to normalise the blood pressure.

Make an infusion of the yellow flowers of wallflower and the leaves of the sorrel and primrose and take two tablespoonfuls per day if your blood pressure is high. If your blood pressure is too low take the same amounts of an infusion of lady's mantle and dandelion in equal measure.

Cooking with salt is supposed to bring out the flavour of the food. It really only brings out the flavour of the salt. A salty diet is harmful to those with blood pressure problems. It is practically impossible in our modern world to devise a salt-free diet — which is just as well as, according to the experts, a totally salt-free diet is dangerous. As everything that goes on a shelf has salt in it, there is rarely any need to add some. The only recommended use for packet salt is as a solution to chimney fires: simply cover the fire with salt, then, most importantly, put the guard up to prevent the burning soot from landing on the carpet.

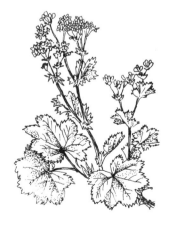

Lady's Mantle

BRONCHITIS

The windpipe divides into two wide tubes, the bronchi, each of which enters one of your lungs, where it divides again into many smaller tubes that carry air into all parts of your lungs. Bronchitis is the result of difficulties encountered by your system in trying to rid itself of toxic substances through the mucous membranes which line the inner surfaces of these tubes. Acute bronchitis is caused either by cold or by the inhalation of fumes, dust or other airborne pollutants. It usually occurs after fevers or rheumatism or as a consequence of heart disease. Congestion of the lungs is followed by bouts of coughing; after some hours the cough softens and relief is obtained. This is known as 'wet' bronchitis. There is a 'dry' variety, in which coughing is very stressful and there is severe pain under the breastbone. If this condition does not clear up quickly, professional assistance is urgently required. Chronic bronchitis may be brought on by a series of bouts of acute bronchitis.

As well as the bronchial tubes, the skin, bowels and kidneys are used to cleanse the body of toxins. Constipation and poor skin conditions are frequently associated with bronchitis. The consumption of superfluous carbohydrate, i.e. sugar and starches, is often a strong contributory factor in bronchitis, if not the original cause. On the positive side, fruit and vegetables eaten as soon as possible after being picked help greatly in the expulsion of toxins. Raw vegetables are best taken as a salad, with free-range eggs, lemon juice and olive oil. Fatty and refined foods, tea, coffee and condiments are all bad for the condition. There are quite palatable substitutes for the dread caffeine, such as dandelion coffee (see 'Dandelion' on page 41). Many herbal infusions will both add interest to your diet and act favourably on bronchitis. These include the teas of the elderflower, meadowsweet, yarrow, angelica, balm, coltsfoot, comfrey and horehound; all should be available from your local health food shop.

To guard against bronchitis, avoid polluted air, take plenty of exercise, eat sensibly (which means sparingly), drink healthful or harmless liquids and maintain your levels of vitamins A and C. Vitamin A is contained in free-range eggs, whole milk, cream cheese, apricots, green leafy vegetables, carrots and fish oils. Vitamin C is found in all green leafy vegetables and in blackberries, blackcurrants, tomatoes, avocados, rose-hip syrup and citrus fruits. All your vitamin levels act together, however, so do not simply binge on a source of one or another.

Carrageen jelly
This is always helpful to sufferers from bronchitis. Take 30 g (1 oz) of carrageen, 600 ml (1 pint) of water, 85 g (3 oz) of honey and two lemons *or* two oranges. Peel the fruit very thinly and add the peel to the water. Bring to the boil and simmer for about quarter of an hour. Strain the juice of the fruit on to the sugar and then strain on the boiling water. Allow to set, decorate and serve.

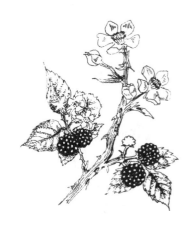

Blackberry

BURNS

Burns and scalds of the first degree are simply those where the damage is near the surface. Although painful, most of these injuries can be successfully treated by the application of any of a number of substances readily available in every kitchen. Second- and third-degree burns are much more serious and generally involve actual wounds or extensive areas of the body. They require immediate medical attention.

A strong element of shock accompanies most burns, however insignificant they seem to be, and the usual treatments of warmth and sweetness should be applied. One of the sweeter herbal teas, say wild blackcurrant or camomile, or a teaspoonful of honey should help in overcoming the trauma. First-degree burns are usually a result of kitchen accidents, and butter, margarine or fat of any kind will very often suffice to avert serious damage. But you should first submerge the burnt part in water for up to half an hour; this excludes the air and reduces the pain. Then take it out and cover it in butter or some other substance — including starch, cream or other milk product, even flour — which is capable of sealing the burnt area against the air. Butter and margarine are the most immediately beneficial and accessible remedies in most kitchens. If, having applied this, you decide that you do not need professional medical attention for the moment, put the burnt part back under water and leave it there until the pain subsides. This will work particularly well with a scald, as I know from experience. I always keep in the kitchen an ointment made from the green inner bark of the elder tree. On one occasion when not attending properly to what I was doing, I managed to pour boiling soup over my hand. I plunged the hand in a bowl of cold water and left it there for almost an hour, then covered it with the ointment and returned it to the water for half an hour. Apart from looking a little redder than my other hand for a day or two, it suffered no ill effects.

In the case of major burns or scalds immerse the burnt area in cool water. If the burn is caused by acid keep it under running water to dilute the acid, then apply bicarbonate of soda. For an extensive burn, cover the area in sheets which have been soaked in cold water and send for medical help. If any clothes become stuck to the burnt area do not remove them without professional help but merely cut the cloth around the area carefully. Administer ointments or lotions with clean hands or, if necessary, with clean cotton cloth but never with any substance like cotton wool which might adhere to the burn.

The inside surface of a houseleek leaf is cool and when applied to a burn will quickly relieve the pain; it will also disinfect and seal the wound. The following ointment made from marigold can then be applied to the burn. Take 600 ml (1 pint) of the leaves, flowers and stems of marigold chopped fine. Heat 450 g (1 lb) of lard until it melts and then stir in the chopped marigold. Remove the pan from the heat, cover and allow to set for a day. The next day warm the mixture until you can strain it through a piece of muslin (into sterilised containers). When not in use, keep the containers sealed. Apply the ointment only with clean hands or on a sterile cloth.

An excellent healing oil for burns is based on St John's Wort. Pick the flowers while the sun is shining, put them in a bottle and cover with linseed oil. Seal the bottle and leave to stand in full sun or beside a source of heat, such as a kitchen stove, for at least a fortnight. When the oil turns red strain it through a muslin cloth and store in brown glass bottles. The linseed oil must be of the variety sold by chemists and not that sold in paint shops.

A follow-up treatment for minor burns which is sometimes used in France is a poultice composed of equal parts of carrots, spinach and cabbage with one ivy leaf, all shredded (a kitchen shredder is perfect for this job). Mix in marigold petals and a little of the juice of nettles. Apply on a clean linen bandage.

A simpler treatment is to soak a cabbage leaf in olive oil for half an hour and then apply it to the burnt part. This is especially appropriate for burns on the hand or arm, which can be immersed in cold water while the poultice is being prepared.

Elder bark ointment for burns is made in the same way as the marigold ointment above.

CATARRH

When the mucous membrane or lining of the throat, nose and sinuses becomes inflamed, usually as the result of a cold, it gives off an increased and toxin-laden mucus which is called catarrh. The body thereby rids itself of poisonous matter which has been accumulating over time and, apart from the inconvenience involved, the process is probably to be welcomed. If you are suffering from catarrh remember that diet plays its usual part in deciding the extent of the problem. The first thing to do is to stop taking milk and, as far as possible, other 'white foods' including white sugar, white flour and, if you can bear it, potatoes. Substitute for these plenty of onions and as much garlic as you can survive socially, raw salads, fresh fruits and green leafy vegetables. Take no fried foods and as little salt as possible and, of course, avoid smoking and smoky atmospheres. Try not to take drugs that suppress the symptoms or you may end up paying an even heavier price in the form of chronic catarrh, which frequently results from retaining the toxins that should have been expelled.

There is a great range of herbs which are beneficial to the condition of catarrh. A professional herbalist would, no doubt, make out a combination to suit your particular variety of catarrh, for there are quite a number of types. But even taken singly and not excessively, many of these herbs can be of advantage, always remem-

bering that no medicine cures you, the true function being to help you, through helping your immune system, to cure yourself.

Two or three tablespoonfuls a day of blackberry syrup is an old country remedy for catarrh; the blackberries should be picked when not fully ripe. A decoction of dried elderflowers is sometimes used as an inhalant for catarrh. A decoction of eucalyptus not alone clears the head when inhaled but also has an expectorant effect. Among herbs to be taken internally is white horehound, an infusion of which will have a generally wholesome and restorative effect. An infusion of ground ivy is not just a first-class expectorant but cleanses the mucous membranes and purges the bowel and kidneys. The nasturtium is a great natural antibiotic which does not have the side-effect of destroying intestinal flora. An infusion of the leaves taken a few times each day should be helpful. Fenugreek tea is used for digestive difficulties occasioned by catarrh.

Three cups a day of an infusion of golden rod will bring relief from catarrh, as will infusions of ground ivy, coltsfoot or comfrey. An infusion of hyssop has a soothing effect while helping to clear the catarrh.

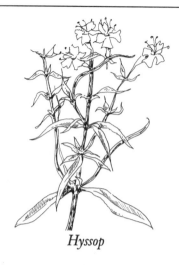

Hyssop

Inhale the vapours from a decoction of camomile flowers. Once the initial heavy perspiration has passed, take a warm infusion of peppermint for a few days; this will maintain a gentle perspiration and combat nausea and general discomfort in the stomach. Be sparing with the heavier foods until health has been restored. If you can, eat onions in raw salads and take plenty of fresh fruit. Lemon juice added to hot water and drunk before breakfast is beneficial.

A syrup made from thyme picked in the sun and layered with honey in a pot is an old remedy for colds and catarrh. Press the layers firmly together and leave the mixture near a source of heat for three to four weeks. Strain through muslin, pressing down well to get as much of the honey as possible through the cloth. Heat gently until it thickens to a syrup. Take an occasional teaspoonful for relief from colds and catarrh.

To get relief from a blocked-up nose, put a few leaves of fresh mint into a bowl and pour boiling water over them. Stand the bowl in your bedroom overnight.

See also 'Common Colds and Chills' below.

COMMON COLDS AND CHILLS

'Never quarrel with a cold,' a naturopathic practitioner once told me, and given that colds clear poisons from the system, you can see what he meant. That feeling of elation when you begin to mend seems to make the having of the cold worth while, and yet how miserable you feel at its onset. Vast has been the research into a cure for the common cold, but it appears that the cold, like the poor, we will always have with us.

Fortunately our experience of colds and chills is long and detailed enough to allow us to make a few ground rules, about both prevention and treatment. We know that if we sit (or drive) in a draught we stand a strong chance of catching a chill; that we are more vulnerable to chills and colds when our general health has run down or been neglected; that if we perspire and then stand about in the cold, the chill may attack us. We also know that sometimes, feeling quite at ease with ourselves and the world, we simply catch cold. When next you feel cold or chilly, whether you are sneezing or shivering or feeling a bit raw in the throat, retreat to your bed with hot drinks of honey and lemon juice, which you should continue to take very frequently. If you haven't got a friend or loved one to keep heating the drinks for you, fill a flask. Above all else, stay warm. Eventually you will perspire, the more freely the better, and your temperature will then return to normal. Forget about work, commitments or social events — the cost of neglect at an early stage could be high.

There is a large number of herbs suitable to the treatment of the common cold in each of its stages. Some are so universally known as hardly to require mention.

Yarrow tea is the best of all to make you sweat it out. An infusion of peppermint and elderblossom in equal parts will achieve much the same purpose. Sage tea is an old remedy for coughs and colds, especially those accompanied by headaches and fevers. It has the additional virtues of being good for the liver and in fact the entire digestive system, helping the body to eliminate waste and toxins. This cannot but assist in overcoming a cold. Sage tea can even be used as a lotion for the skin, and this too will facilitate excretion of the toxic substances which are part and parcel of colds. For relief of the nasal passages and sinuses inhale the fumes of grated horseradish. If you don't have a piece of horseradish root to hand, get a jar of horseradish sauce, remove the lid and inhale gently.

Inhale the vapours from a warm decoction of eucalyptus leaves or camomile flowers. Make a tea out of equal parts of balm, angelica and peppermint and take it freely. An old country cure is an onion sliced and simmered in milk or water. Season it with cayenne pepper and take it as a warming soup. Borage, hyssop and agrimony in equal quantities taken as a tea have long been employed for breaking up a cold. A quarter-teaspoonful of ground ginger in hot water with a spoon or two of honey is one of the more enjoyable drinks to relieve a cold. Drinking thyme tea regularly in the autumn months is said to protect you from colds during the following winter.

See also 'Catarrh', page 112.

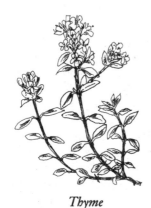

Thyme

CONSTIPATION

Constipation is most often caused by dietary deficiencies, when it is not part of some other ailment. It is, by and large, a condition of the sedentary life and is probably more common nowadays when people do not exert themselves physically as much as in former times. Persistent constipation is a most debilitating problem and brings with it headaches, abdominal pains and haemorrhoids.

The main dietary cause of constipation is the absence of suitable fibre in the diet. Refined foods are once again the villains of the piece. Before breakfast eat half a dozen prunes, steeped overnight in warm water with a teaspoonful of blackstrap molasses. Wholegrain breakfast foods should be taken instead of refined ones; salads and raw vegetables will also help. Linseed may be added to the cereal in the morning or a dessertspoonful may be taken with a glass of water before you go to bed (the water will stop the seeds sticking in your mouth). Liquorice root is gentle with a pleasing taste, and a decoction can be effective.

Ask yourself if you are not eating too much of everything. The extra slice of bread and the occasional extra potato or apple stretch one's digestive powers beyond their limits. Eating too fast is a major cause of constipation; another – rarely suspected – is tea. Tea is a diuretic. It promotes urination and so deprives your system of moisture which is needed to facilitate the proper digestion of food. If you are a serious tea drinker and constipated, try cutting back your consumption; you should soon notice an improvement. There are many purges, herbal and otherwise, which treat constipation, but examining your diet, intake of liquid and general habits —

including exercise — will often suggest simple courses of action that are quite as effective, and definitely less stressful.

A recipe book of the early nineteenth century contains the following remedy for constipation. Mash well together 110 g (¼ lb) each of stoneless raisins and of figs and add 55 g (2 oz) of senna powder (available from chemists' shops) and a teaspoonful of powdered ginger. Roll up the mixture like a Swiss roll and take a thin slice each day until relief is obtained. Keep the roll wrapped in greaseproof paper and in a covered jar.

A gentle laxative which is easy to make up and to take consists of 80 to 90 g (a few ounces) of liquorice root brought to the boil in 1.1 litres (1 quart) of cold water and allowed to simmer for ten minutes. Cool and strain the decoction and have a cupful two or three times a day. This remedy has the recommendation of placing minimal stress on the system.

Porridge and wholegrain cereal are preferable to the rather insipid and sugary substitutes foisted on the public through mass advertising.

Yoghurt with mashed apricots and honey mixed in is another easy way to ensure that children, in particular, remain healthy and free from constipation. A shredded apple in place of the apricots would help to achieve the same purpose, especially when a light sprinkling of bran is added. For an interesting salad dressing and dip which is straightforward to make and should have the desired effect, grate a dessert apple and a very little horseradish, mix with a little lemon juice and a tablespoonful of yoghurt or sour cream.

An infusion of rose-hips, carefully strained, makes a pleasant drink which is mildly laxative. Among the gentler laxatives which can be taken in standard infusions are couch grass rhizomes (see 'Couch Grass', page 38), sage, the leaves of the redcurrant (*Ribes rubrum*) and the shoots of fennel.

DEPRESSION

Depression is undoubtedly frequently linked to general health problems which may not seem immediately relevant. We all know the expressions 'He is in a liver', or 'His bile has been aroused', and though these happen to refer to fits of bad temper, they make the point that the state of the mind is often reflected in the state of the body and vice versa.

Without getting into the endless discussion about which goes wrong first, the body or the mind, there was something in the old Roman motto about a healthy mind requiring a healthy body. There are, alas, depressions for which no cure is known. But the condition can very often be alleviated if its causes are properly diagnosed and the appropriate measures applied.

Low or neglected general health following severe or prolonged illness or childbirth often causes depression. Proper nutrition and recuperative rest contribute significantly to the restoration of normal spirits in many such cases. Among the herbal or dietary aids to recovery of health and strength, blackstrap molasses takes an important place. It is a great blood tonic and can make a very pleasant nightcap, taken in warmed, but not hot, milk. Borage has enjoyed a reputation as a restorer of good spirits since ancient times. Its leaves should be taken in infusion twice a day, especially when going to bed. There is a school of thought which traces depression and other weaknesses of mind to disorders of the kidneys. Both stinging nettle and yarrow taken as tea are said to improve the state of the kidneys and thus, in at least some

cases, combat the depression. Horsetail tea is also recommended. These teas, drunk even occasionally, should have a cheering effect on the sufferer, provided that attention is paid to general diet. Allergy can be a cause, or a contributory cause, of depression and it would be worth the time and trouble to have a comprehensive allergy test.

Four or five of the flowering spikes of lavender to a cupful of boiling water with a little honey added makes a good antidote to depression when strained and taken cool. The leaves of bog myrtle prepared in a standard infusion can be of assistance. Honegar, apple cider vinegar and honey mixed, in a glass of slightly warmed water should be taken night and morning. Chervil used to flavour salads has a cheering effect. Lemon balm, vervain, camomile and valerian taken individually or together in equal proportions in an infusion raise the spirits. An infusion of speedwell taken before going to bed is reputedly beneficial; mixed with celery roots, the speedwell is an even more powerful antidote to depression.

Steep a bucketful of St John's Wort, flowers, leaves and stems, in cold water overnight. Boil everything the following morning and add it to a bath. Soak in the bath for about half an hour. To prevent yourself from falling asleep leave the radio on in another room and sing along. This bath will help you to overcome the worst symptoms of depression. Two hundred and twenty-five grams (½ lb) of dried thyme prepared in the same way and added to the morning bath should have a similar effect.

DIARRHOEA

This ailment can strike suddenly and leave you feeling devastated — or not leave you and render you desperate for a quick cure. Very often its causes are mysterious: a change of location, say going on holiday, can trigger an attack. We seem to be especially vulnerable to changes in our drinking water. Many people bring water with them on holidays or buy bottled and supposedly uncontaminated water for the duration of their stay, but it often happens that if they even wash their teeth in the local water they are smitten by the 'bugs'.

Nutrients, vitamins, body fluids and minerals are taken out of the body by diarrhoea. Loss of sodium leaves you feeling weak, so add a little salt to your (boiled) drinking water and eat salty foods to restore you. Two teaspoons of cider vinegar added to every glass of water you drink can be a marvellous aid to recovery; bacteria cannot survive in an acid medium. I never travel without cider vinegar and, in fact use it freely at home also. Public water supplies, especially in summer, cannot be guaranteed to be immune from harmful intrusions. Teaspoonfuls of the cider vinegar/water taken at five-minute intervals for half an hour followed by three or four glasses of the mixture at half-hourly intervals are reputed to have cured bad cases of diarrhoea.

Food poisoning is sometimes the cause of very severe diarrhoea. Unripe fruit can be another culprit, and allergy to various foods. Then there is chemical pollution of our food-chain, which is increasing as a source of stomach trouble in our high-tech environment. Where at all possible, food should be thoroughly washed before being cooked to remove chemical residues.

Among the many herbal aids to overcoming diarrhoea, cayenne pepper or capsicum is an old favourite. It will kill the parasites in the intestine which sometimes cause the diarrhoea. Camomile tea is known to have stopped the disease in its tracks, and honey is capable of killing germs and makes a natural accompaniment to cider vinegar. Live yoghurt and other acidified milk products are recognised as controllers of both diarrhoea and dysentery. If you are given an antibiotic by a doctor be sure to take live yoghurt with it; antibiotics kill good 'bugs' as well as bad but live yoghurt helps to restore the balance. An alternative to live yoghurt here is acidophilus, available in health food shops. When you have finished taking the antibiotic, take a short course of brewer's yeast tablets.

To help you overcome the dehydration which is usually the worst effect associated with diarrhoea, take liberal quantities of the following mixture: 1 litre (1¾ pints) of freshly boiled water to two tablespoons of honey, a quarter-teaspoon of bicarbonate of soda, a quarter-teaspoon of sea salt and a dash of lemon juice. Have a little every five minutes so that you will have taken 3 litres (5¼ pints) in twenty-four hours. One litre (1¾ pints) will do for children.

Foods which aid recuperation include a watery gruel of oatmeal, plain live yoghurt, boiled rice, and a little banana.

An infusion of blackberry roots with a little powdered

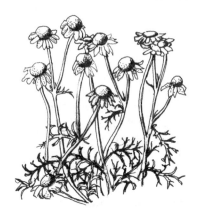

Camomile

ginger or cinnamon also assists recovery. A standard infusion of agrimony is particularly useful for diarrhoea in children, who should drink one cup three times a day. A very safe infusion for children is made with coriander, a spice which can be obtained in grocery shops and supermarkets. An infusion of Self-heal (*Prunella vulgaris*) taken three times daily will have a healing effect. Marigold tea sometimes helps to clear up a lingering case of diarrhoea.

DIGESTIVE DISORDERS

There is a great variety of digestive disorders and an even greater variety of 'cures', effective and otherwise. Lacking the space here to cover the subject in detail, I will concentrate on a few of the more common forms of digestive disfunction and some of the tried and tested antidotes. However, if any of these symptoms persists see your medical practitioner.

Hippocrates' saying, which I keep returning to, is perhaps most relevant here: 'Let your medicine be your food and your food your medicine.' The entire range of culinary herbs will assist your digestion when taken with meals. Whether it be ham seasoned with juniper or liver cooked with sage leaves, the benefit of cooking with herbs is beyond question. Thyme, garlic, parsley, marjoram, lemon and onions are marvellous stuffing for game and poultry. Fennel and dill take the harm out of baked oily fish. Horseradish makes beef digestible as well as killing intestinal parasites, including the tapeworm which afflicts serious beef eaters.

But particular disagreeable conditions of the digestion can also be safely and easily alleviated by appropriate herbs taken alone or in combination. Apple cider vinegar added regularly to your drinking water should rid you of heartburn or acidity. Even simply drinking water in liberal quantities will dilute the acid and make you feel better. A stem of angelica chewed slowly should rid you of stom-ach pains which originate in digestive difficulties — but don't confuse angelica with the poisonous hemlock which it resembles. Five or six cloves taken in infusion will cope with flatulence. My own favourite is fennel, which never fails to settle even the most turbulent and painful rumblings of wind in the stomach. A fennel plant looks well in any garden and a few fronds picked, washed and taken as a tisane refresh and relieve almost instantaneously. Fengugreek tea is used for digestive problems occasioned by catarrh.

Apart from herbs there are many old and trusted natural antidotes to digestive troubles. Yoghurt is a great soother of sick stomachs. Soda water is known to remedy flatulence and is most refreshing when taken after travelling. Charcoal tablets are good for nausea, heartburn and wind.

An infusion of equal parts of dandelion, catmint, agrimony and camomile is a useful aid to digestion, as is an infusion of golden rod. Acquire some powdered bark of slippery elm (available at chemists), mix a tablespoonful with cold water and add to a cup of hot milk. Drink at night before going to bed.

One tablespoonful of ground aniseed boiled in a cup

of milk taken a few times a day will help the digestive processes; so will hot peppermint tea after a meal. Take horseradish with beef, rosemary with fat lamb and fennel with oily fish. Take goats' milk for continuing heartburn, charcoal biscuits or tablets for the same and also for nausea. Take oats or porridge for flatulence, garlic for general digestion and to prevent food poisoning, and cook your meat with marjoram if you are inclined to indigestion. Make aniseed tea for heartburn. The dandelion root aids digestion so substitute dandelion coffee for the usual coffee after meals. Above all, take your time eating.

Another cure for indigestion consists of warming 300 ml (½ pint) of milk in a saucepan with a pinch of nutmeg and a pinch of pepper. Warm it well but do not allow it to boil. A little honey may be added for taste. Drink it warm.

Earache

Vigorous blowing of the nose drives infection through the Eustachian tubes and creates the conditions for earache. Small children are particularly prone to earache owing to the narrowness of their undeveloped tubes, which easily become blocked and painful. Warm a little oil of almonds or olive oil and put a few drops in the ear. Do not heat the oil, simply take the chill off it. A few warm drops of either hyssop or yarrow infusion should have the same effect. The juice of the coltsfoot, freshly pressed, is another treatment for earache. If the drum of the ear has suffered damage, do not put drops of oil or lotion in it.

There is an old country cure which is said to do wonders for earache. Put your feet in a basin of very hot water and simultaneously apply cold wet compresses to the back of your neck. Go on doing this for as long as it takes to stop the earache. This sounds a bit daft but it may just work — though how or why, I have no idea. Maybe the shock of the hot feet and cold head creates an alternative set of sensations to worry about and takes your mind off the earache. Napoleon used to say that if you have trouble at home you should start a foreign war.

Another odd-sounding theory has it that a middle finger inserted loosely in the ear and rotated, in one direction then the other, gives some kind of magnetic treatment to the ear. It goes on to stipulate that the hand should remain clenched and parallel with the ground, and should not be that of the sufferer but that of a friend. It is, of course, frequently said that you should put nothing smaller than your elbow in your ear. You pays your money and you takes your pick. At least, in its favour, the elbow theory draws our attention to the extreme sensitivity of the ear.

Tinnitus, or noises in the ear, can have many causes: high blood pressure, anaemia and fatigue, to name a few. Garlic has the double effect of clearing catarrh and of lowering blood pressure and is sometimes beneficial to the sufferer from tinnitus.

Sage, dandelion, onion, hawthorn and broom all help to regulate the circulation of the blood. In doing so they often relieve the condition known as 'ringing in the ears'. Steep hands and feet in 1 litre (1¾ pints) of water to which hawthorn leaves, sage and dandelion flowers, roots and leaves have been added.

ECZEMA

With eczema we are into the notoriously complex area of allergies, and yet the experts say that eczema is less a disease of the skin than a symptom of some internal problem, usually in the bowel. Some eczemas are very quickly cured when an allergy is discovered and its sources removed. Cows' milk allergy is a case in point, where a change to goats' milk is usually enough to heal the condition. Many claims are made for goats' milk in relation to other allergies. This is not surprising as goats feed on practically the entire of nature's pharmacy and are reputed to be entirely free from brucellosis. Their milk is healthy and nourishing and certainly worth a try in any allergic problem; even if not the solution, it will have a generally beneficial effect on the sufferer — unless, of course, he or she is allergic to goats' milk. A friend of mine was diagnosed, in a most respectable medical establishment, as being allergic to camels. I did not dare to suggest that he was a case for healing by pyramid power.

A few tablespoonfuls of safflower oil taken internally at the rate of two teaspoonfuls per day will have a beneficial effect in some cases of eczema where the skin is dry and scaly. Various vitamin deficiencies are at least partly to blame for some of the forms of eczema with which people are afflicted. The skin is an organ of elimination for poisons in the system, but it should only be expected to do its fair share. It develops all manner of abnormalities when required to do the work of the bowel in clearing toxic substances from the body, so constipation should be avoided by anyone suffering from eczema. Half an apple or a potato rubbed on itchy skin is sometimes helpful. Never scratch but instead brush itchy skin with a soft brush (available in health food and chemists' shops). An old cure for eczema is to take honey and vinegar with meals, a teaspoonful of each in a glass of water sipped while eating, and apply diluted cider vinegar to the skin as frequently as necessary. A medical herbalist and/or a dietitian should be of particular assistance to eczema sufferers as both specialise in the relationship between the human metabolism and the world of things organic; and the causes of eczema seem to lie in complex malfunctions or disruptions in what should be an harmonious relationship between plants (and food) and man.

Hang a muslin bag containing one cupful of flake oatmeal under the hot tap when you are filling the bath, and leave the bag in the water while you are bathing. This should ease the discomfort of eczema and dry skin.

A strained infusion of plantain leaves makes an agreeable lotion for the affected parts. The following herbs help to keep the skin free of eczema in whatever form they are taken: chicory, cabbage, burdock, carrot, artichoke, briar, broom, bilberry, sage, rose, turnip and nettle. Pulp the cabbage leaves and drink the juice. Eat the carrots raw, drink their juice or grate them and make a poultice. Eat watercress and use its juice as a lotion. A handful of cabbage leaves, a handful of artichoke leaves and a handful of celandine leaves, infused in 2 litres (3½ pints) of water and allowed to cool will make a lotion which may be of use. The juice of the strawberry is reputed to clear eczema; a lotion made from an infusion of the leaves can be equally healing to the skin and is also said to remedy styes.

Look for slippery elm soap in your chemist or health food shop. The juice of chickweed makes an effective lotion. A poultice of crushed linseed, which is good for psoriasis and shingles, may also be of some benefit.

EMPHYSEMA

Emphysema consists of a chronic distension of the

air-sacs in the lungs. It is brought on by chronic bronchitis or asthma, by working in conditions which demand strenuous breathing, possibly even by over-energetic blowing of musical wind instruments. With emphysema the air gets trapped in the sacs and cannot be expelled as quickly as it should be. The more pressure that is put on the lungs, the greater the tendency for these sacs to inflate when they should actually be deflating. This leads to weakness, as in the membrane of an over-inflated balloon, and finally to the collapse of the sacs. Emphysema can also be caused by upward pressure on heart, bronchial tubes and lungs from a swollen liver. The disease is said to be irreversible in its later stages; however, the starting-point of the discussion should really be, as with all diseases, that an ounce of prevention is worth more than a ton of cure.

It is most important for parents to realise that drinks from the refrigerator can give children bronchitis, which in turn can eventually lead to emphysema. The child's bronchial tubes and entire system are comparatively tender, and the sudden application of freezing liquid can shock and possibly seriously damage the sensitive mucous membrane, or interior skin, of these tubes. Slightly warmed drinks are always more appropriate and more refreshing in hot weather.

A decoction of comfrey root, liquorice root and crushed aniseed can be very helpful in this complaint as it will tend to heal the inflamed passages. The diet should be such as to discourage the excessive production of mucous and the usual injunction against white foods applies. Fresh raw fruit, salads and vegetables assist the bowel to perform its function of elimination efficiently, thereby taking the strain off the lungs.

The leaves and flowers of the mallow added to barley soup are beneficial to emphysema sufferers. Another, more effective application of the herb is to soak the flowers and leaves overnight in cold water in order to retain the mucilage. Strain off the water, infuse the mallow and allow to cool. Drink a slightly warmed cupful three times during the day. Strain and warm the leaves and flowers and apply to the chest as a poultice overnight.

GALLSTONES

We are back to our old friend the diet again, in this case with a vengeance. Cholesterol and bile salts form gallstones, and they are almost entirely the product of wrong living. Overeating of rich foods and lack of exercise are the main culprits. This is the original life-style disease and can only be permanently eliminated by a change in habits.

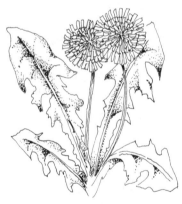

Dandelion

In the meantime, life must go on — and life can be made miserable indeed by the discomfort of gallstones. Try the dandelion for some relief. Collect the leaves before the plant flowers and take them in salads. When the flowers come on, eat the stems, which should remove the gallstones without making you suffer in the process. Make dandelion coffee (see 'Dandelions', page 41). The dandelion brings other benefits to health; it purifies the blood, stimulates the digestion, and improves the condition of the skin. A syrup made from the flowers is quite pleasant, despite its slight bitterness; add honey to taste. The neglected dandelion is one of our strongest natural allies in the constant battle against disease.

The juice of radishes, taken over a period, can often dissolve gallstones (it can be satisfactorily acquired by putting the radishes in an ordinary extractor). Start by taking one tablespoonful and increase gradually for two to three weeks until you are taking four tablespoonfuls and then, over another two to three weeks, bring the dose back down to one tablespoonful. This radish juice is fairly hot stuff, so be careful that it doesn't inflame the lining of your stomach. A few spoons of honey taken between doses should help. If you do feel uncomfortable don't panic, just cut back on the juice. A little of it goes a long way, as with all herbal applications. When you have rid yourself of the gallstones, take an occasional small shot of radish juice, and go for regular walks. Hippocrates was right: we have two physicians, Doctor Left Foot and Doctor Right. And walk away from, rather than towards, the confectionery shop.

A teaspoonful of olive oil and a few drops of lemon juice taken before each meal should bring a certain amount of relief from pain. An extended version of this remedy is said to remove gallstones altogether and can be discussed in detail with either your herbalist or medical practitioner.

A standard infusion of the violet (*Viola odorata*) is reputed to be one of nature's most powerful dissolvents and has been generally used in the past for the removal of stones.

GOUT

Gout is another life-style disease, usually brought on by over-indulgence in rich foods, meat and alcohol. It affects the joint of the big toe, which becomes very painful. The first thing to do, obviously, is to cut out the offending foods and drink. Change to health-giving leafy vegetables and include lots of parsley in your menu. In fact, the nearer you can reasonably go to a strictly vegetarian diet the better, but only while the condi-

tion lasts. There are so many herbal remedies for gout as to be almost countless. A short list will have to suffice for our present purpose.

As the immediate cause of gout is a build-up of uric acid in the system, parsley tea is a good way to start the cure. A tea made from the butterbur or umbrella plant (*Petasites officinalis*) is also helpful. The cowslip (*Primula officinalis*) is said to rid the blood of the offending substances which bring on gout. A four-week course of dandelion flower-stems (eat six per day) is an old remedy for gout, and a cup of horsetail tea (*Equisetum arvense*) taken daily is supposed to work wonders. An infusion of speedwell is also said to be very effective and our good friend the stinging nettle taken as a tea will also help greatly. A compress of comfrey (*Symphytum officinale*) on the afflicted toe will bring down the swelling and ease the pain. This compress can be made either with fresh grated root or with the powder of the dried root. The leaves of mint (*Mentha*) fresh or dried can also be made into a compress for the toe. An unguent of sage, using the leaves, contributes to recovery when rubbed into the toe-joint. A balm of St John's Wort has the advantage that it can be made and stored against the day when gout might strike.

Take broom tops, meadowsweet, dandelion root and burdock root in equal quantities, leave in cold water for a few hours, bring to the boil and simmer for two minutes, then infuse for half an hour before straining. Drink a wineglassful before each meal.

A poultice of bran and vinegar or of garlic and tallow brings relief to the affected toe. So does a flannel cloth soaked in honey or a poultice of hot cabbage leaves. Apples, onions and pears should become part of the diet, as should all or any of the following: artichoke, blackcurrant, camomile, dandelion, sage, thyme and rosemary.

Celery boiled in milk and added to the diet may bring results and is worth taking anyway for its own sake.

Beware, having finally cured yourself of this so-called 'rich man's disease': the Inland Revenue may be waiting to question you as to how you acquired such an expensive disease in the first instance.

HAEMORRHOIDS

These are veins in the anus which become swollen because of some pressure. They can be caused by pregnancy or constipation or even by congestion of the liver. If pregnancy is the cause consult a gynaecologist. Otherwise the application of some astringent should suffice to shrink the swollen veins and relieve the suffering involved. This suffering can take the form of either itching and heat in the rectum if the haemorrhoids are internal, or pain and a feeling of pressure if they are external.

Life-style and diet have a great deal to do with this complaint. Hours spent sitting at the wheel of a car, interspersed with heavy, stodgy feeding, are a recipe for piles, as the condition is usually called. In the long term, attention to diet and exercise is the most important means of countering haemorrhoids, but in the meantime try applying an ointment made from the root of the lesser celandine or pilewort, known as a remedy from at least Anglo-Saxon times. Wort is the Anglo-Saxon word for 'root', and 'pile' is self-explanatory. This ointment should be applied after bowel movements and at least three times a day. An infusion of blackberry leaves or cranesbill will help if taken internally. If constipation is causing the problem, examine your diet to see if you are short of fibre. To encourage bowel action try linseed, which can be bought in any health food shop. (Buy it loose rather than in packets as it is much more economical.) Mix it with porridge or other breakfast cereal, or take a dessertspoonful with a glass of water before going to bed. Eat nuts and salads and lots of fruit and take a forty-minute walk once a day — perhaps every second day to begin with, as a sudden change from laziness to exercise can briefly accentuate constipation. Don't drink tea, coffee or any diuretic as they will dry your bowel and impede elimination. Drink plenty of water. Avoid conventional laxatives as they frequently do more harm than good. Smoking has a drying effect on your entire system and can be a contributory cause of constipation and therefore of piles.

The New Era tissue salt labelled combination G (available at chemists' and health food shops) is well worth a try, having been used by some people with spectacular success. Another remedy credited with almost instant success is the B complex of vitamins, especially B6. Don't take B6 on its own, though; take it at the same time as the other B vitamins.

To make ointment from the pilewort, or lesser celandine (*Ranunculus ficaria*) dig the roots in spring and pound them together with an equal weight of lard. Allow them to macerate for five days in a glass or stoneware jar. Heat gently and press through a cloth. Administer externally.

A decoction of yarrow can be used as a compress or honey can be applied.

HALITOSIS/BAD BREATH

Bad breath can be caused by any of a number of complaints. It can even be caused by choking the underarm sweat glands with certain commercial products, thereby transferring the duty of expelling toxic substances to the lungs. Think twice before applying any of these products on your way to the disco; the same person who didn't dance with you for one reason may keep even further away from you for another. Tooth decay, eating substandard food or highly flavoured food like garlic are among the more common causes of bad breath; cheese is another. Diseases of the sinus, throat and mouth can give rise to bad breath, as can constipation.

So what to do? To begin with, if there is an underlying cause like constipation or tooth decay, rectify it and your breath should automatically come right. If in the meantime you wish to disguise the foul smell, chew a piece of mint or a few seeds of fennel, cloves, aniseed or even parsley. All have a cleansing effect on your breath, especially if you have just eaten strongly flavoured food. (Parsley is said to be particularly effective at dispelling the odour of garlic.) If a sore throat is the root of the trouble, try a little honey and lemon in slightly warmed water or, even better, a teaspoonful of cider vinegar, also in warm water. Gargle for as long as you can and then swallow. This recommendation to swallow may shock you but it is soundly based, for the bacteria which cause the infection almost invariably lie well below the area reached by gargling. Use something you feel happy about swallowing — like cider vinegar — and not some patent antiseptic that tastes like a paint remover. Don't drink water while eating as this confuses your gastric juices. Syrup of figs is an old and tried remedy for the condition; take a teaspoon in a glass of hot water before going to bed. Worms cause bad breath in children.

Peppermint in infusion can be taken for bad breath which arises from digestive upsets. A mouthwash made with sea salt and bread soda in water will clear the breath. So will rose-mary, thyme, marjoram or lavender, or all four combined with vinegar; dilute with water and use as a mouthwash. An infusion of lemon verbena is also recommended. Unless the problem is a serious one, however, it is easiest simply to chew any of the above herbs.

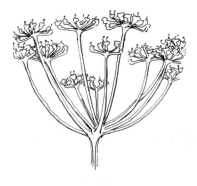

Fennel

HEADACHE

Trying to list the possible causes for headache almost gives one a headache, which makes the point that you oughtn't to panic if you get an unexplained headache, unless of course it persists for a fairly long time and recurs. A short list of causes could include con-cussion, tension, various things to do with teeth, gums and sinuses, constipation, bad digestion, fatigue, difficulties relating to periods and, of course, emotional stresses of one kind or another. Concussion is always potentially serious and a matter for professional medical observation. Eye-strain can cause headache and so can that same old collection of hardy annuals: alcohol taken to excess, dairy products, caffeine as in coffee or tea, and tobacco smoke, whether actively or passively imbibed. Even the scent of certain exotic flowers can cause headache. Gardenia and heliotrope affect some people, and lilac is said to be a particular culprit.

There are many herbal remedies for headache. However, it is always best before applying a remedy (except in some emergency like a burn) to try to work out what the cause of the complaint might be. Have you been sitting before the computer VDU for several hours together? Are you badly constipated? Have you fallen and struck your head? Even if you take herbal or any other cures, do not neglect to tackle the real cause; if you don't, then don't blame the herbs if the problem recurs.

The leaves of any of the following herbs, if crushed in your hand and their scents inhaled, will go a long way towards clearing your head: violet, peppermint, rose, lavender, sage, dill and lemon balm. (I mention only those most commonly found in a garden.) A cut lemon applied to the temple is an ancient cure for headache. Crush some rosemary leaves and put them in 300 ml (½ pint) of olive oil, seal and leave in a warm atmosphere for two to three weeks. Rub the resulting liquid on your temples when the headache comes. Inhale the fumes of heated malt vinegar, or add it to herbal teas like camomile (a little should be effective). The very best way to relieve headache, according to some authorities, is to have your feet massaged, especially at the joints between your toes and your foot. Even a footbath could ease the pain.

Sleep with your head on a pillow stuffed with lavender and drink an infusion of the flowers of lavender two or three times per day. Float a few fragrant rose petals on a bowl of warmed water to which two tablespoons of malt vinegar have been added and leave it in your bedroom overnight.

HEART DISEASES

The heart can be affected in so many ways that it is possible here only to make a few comments about this, the most important organ of all. I have already discussed anaemia and it is sufficient to say that good, clean, healthy blood has a bearing on the general state of health of the heart. Liver, kidney and lung actions also influence the heart's efficiency ; so do digestion, the thyroid gland and, intangibly but most significantly, the state of the mind. Any drug which either suppresses or stimulates the functioning of the system has a potentially detrimental effect on the heart. Tea, coffee, alcohol and, of course, tobacco all fall into the category of stimulant. Remember that every 'upper' is followed by a 'downer'. If you cheer yourself up with a cup of coffee and a cigarette, you will soon need another 'fix' as you will have come down further than you have gone up. We owe to journalist and Women's Lib pioneer Erin Pizzey the first articulate description of adrenalin addiction. This most insidious of conditions arises especially in those activities which take place in a state of great excitement. We get a shot of adrenalin to help us in our heightened reactions to the crises of life, reactions which usually take the form of either 'fight' or 'flight'. All of this is quite natural. The trouble arises when we grow addicted to the feeling of well-being which the adrenalin gives us as an aid to, and compensation for, surviving in this dangerous world. We then expose ourselves to exciting situations purely for the sake of the adrenalin, in the process wearing ourselves out and placing unnecessary and destructive pressure on our blood-circulatory systems and on our hearts. Cigarette smoking is a form of adrenalin addiction. There are many, many more. Is there any form of excitement in your life which you suspect yourself of enjoying too much? If there is, then to that extent you are adrenalin addicted.

Animal fats and dairy products do not promote heart health. Neither does high-protein or high-salt eating. Your doctor will supply you with details of the diet largely agreed as being good for your heart. Herbs that are taken for the heart include hawthorn, which lowers the blood pressure while it strengthens the heart muscle, and foxglove (by medical prescription only), which corrects arrhythmia and improves the action of the heart. Heart disease is a challenge that frequently spurs people to amend their life-styles in time to have a sometimes surprisingly healthy old age. It need not be a killer. But watch the adrenalin. Speak to your yoga friends about techniques for keeping your emotions under control. Ask your doctor about combining herbs with medications. If you think he or she simply doesn't know the answers ask a herbalist or homeopath. Remember that certain herbs taken intelligently are part of normal diet, but some herbs are obviously more definite in their effects than others. Combine sound advice with your own body's reactions to arrive at whatever suits your particular condition.

The treatment of heart disorders has become so highly technical that it is impossible in a book like this to discuss it. All one can do is to re-emphasise the life-style origins of most of the heart problems which are afflicting our stress-ridden, overfed and underexercised generation. To feel guilty about any of these three cardinal sins is both counter-productive and unrealistic — it is more the time we live in that is at fault. Blame the age for the prevalence of heart disease, then, but make the necessary changes in your own life-style to preserve you from a disease which you can probably avoid.

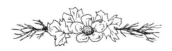

INSOMNIA

Insomnia can scarcely be called a life-threatening disease and, perhaps for this reason, it is frequently not taken too seriously, except by those whom it affects. There can be many reasons for insomnia, varying from a bad conscience to irregular habits acquired in childhood. The good news is that it can be alleviated. It would be foolish to say 'cured' as even a few restless nights might unduly upset insomnia sufferers who were on the way to normal sleep patterns and discourage them from persisting in their remedial efforts.

It often angers people who suffer from insomnia to be told by 'experts' that they really sleep far more than they imagine. The anger is understandable although there is sometimes a grain of truth in what the experts say. But it's best to ignore such contentious matters lest they be the causes of even more serious insomnia — there's nothing like a good grievance for keeping you awake. Better then to concentrate on positive suggestions on how to cope with the problem.

Exercise before bedtime can have a salutary effect. A good brisk walk is among the great inducers of sleep. This is attended by some difficulties in our time. There's not much point in trying to solve insomnia by being put to sleep by a mugger, and if you dig the garden late at night you're being unfair, not just to the birds but to the worms as well — not to mention the neighbours. Many praise a warm bath with a bunch of hops in a muslin bag added to the water. It makes you luxuriously drowsy. But don't fall asleep in the bath. Drowning may be more comfortable than being mugged, but it's still not the answer. Going to bed too late and too tired can prevent you from sleeping properly. Television watching has become a major source of insomnia in our time — and indeed also of nightmares — and this effect is worsening with the ever-increasing violence which is part and parcel, not alone of contemporary films, but even of TV news bulletins. Turn off the television early in the evening, listen round-eyed to soothing music, take a little warm milk with blackstrap molasses and say a little prayer for a troubled world. Incidentally, if you do get nightmares, try a sprig of rosemary under your pillow; it is supposed to give you sweet dreams.

There are many herbal infusions said to be good for insomnia, and there are many which are definitely not. The ones that will help include limeblossom tea, camomile tea and an infusion in equal parts of hops, valerian and passiflora.

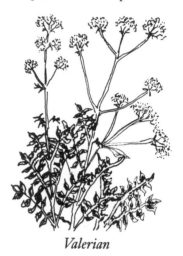

Valerian

This last infusion you should drink cold. Onions have a restorative effect on your nerves. The herb teas which you should not drink are the strongly diuretic ones as they will wake you to answer the call of nature at various times during the night and thus disturb the pattern of your sleep. Indian tea is a diuretic and will have this effect. If you have been on medication your nerves may be suffering from calcium depletion, which can cause loss of sleep. Take a calcium lactate tablet a few times a day to remedy this deficiency.

Your chemist or health food shop will have many herbal preparations for you to try in turn until your sleep pattern is restored to normal.

KIDNEY DISEASES

It is always necessary to have kidney problems looked after by a medical practitioner but herbal preparations can play an important part in relieving many kidney complaints and can probably even prevent certain of them from arising in the first place. Water which contains fluoride or even any kind of 'hard' or limey water places a strain on the kidneys and is best avoided because of the danger of kidney stones. There are many herbal means of dissolving kidney stones but it is obviously more desirable to prevent them from forming.

Among the many herbs which are stimulating to the kidneys, the dandelion is surely the best and gentlest. It can be taken in many forms — as a coffee, a tea, and as an ingredient in a salad. The tender young leaves taken in spring will be found to have a general tonic effect. If you blanch them (by placing an upturned bucket over the plant for a few days before you pluck the leaves), they should taste less bitter.

Horsetail will help to dissolve the stone while agrimony will tone up the mucous membrane or 'inner skin' of the entire urinary system. Parsley is the age-old remedy for many conditions of the kidney and has a generally beneficial effect on the system.

The blackcurrant (*Ribes nigrum*) is one of the most famous of herbal cures for many kidney complaints: sufferers from gravel, retention of urine, inflammation of the urinary system (including cystitis), dropsy and renal colic all benefit by taking blackcurrant leaves in infusion. If you are using the dried leaves let them soak for an hour in cold water, boil them gently, remove from the heat and let them infuse for ten minutes. In equal parts with liquorice, say one teaspoonful of each to 1 litre (1¾ pints) of water, they will make a marvellous diuretic. The blackcurrant has traditionally been esteemed as a source of longevity.

Golden rod (*Solidago virgaurea*), drunk either as a decoction or a syrup, stimulates the action of the kidneys and promotes the elimination of impurities. However, it should not be taken for more than eight days at a time followed by a rest period of eight days, otherwise you may tire the kidneys. The onion is a marvellous aid to general health and in no case is it more effective than with the kidney. If you can possibly eat it raw, perhaps finely chopped in salads, all the better. As an alternative, put four medium-sized onions in 1 litre (1¾ pints) of hot water and allow to macerate for two to three hours. Strain and drink the resulting liquid. You will find no better tonic for the kidneys.

Herbs which when eaten are beneficial to the kidneys are runner beans, parsley and watercress. Asparagus and melon are also useful, and beetroot has a tendency to dissolve kidney stones. Strong cider taken daily will dissolve kidney stones. It may also turn you into an alcoholic. Parsnips and their juice, and the sloe, or fruit of the blackthorn, will all help to dissolve the stones.

The Hippocratic kidney tonic is an ancient cure made up of equal parts of violet, groundsel or meadowsweet, fennel, eyebright and nettle or parsley, made into an infusion and taken cold at the rate of two tablespoonfuls a day.

Barley water is an old and well-known cure for kidney ailments. Take three tablespoonfuls of barley, one lemon (sliced) and 1.7 litres (3 pints) of water. Wash the barley in warm water. Put into a pot with the water and the lemon and simmer gently until the liquid is reduced by half. Strain and cool. A little honey may be added if wished. A half-cupful before breakfast and another before going to bed was supposed to be a marvellous tonic for weak kidneys.

For another useful tonic boil 30 g (1 oz) of couch grass root in 900 ml (1½ pints) of water for five minutes. Strain and take a half-cupful four times per day.

LIVER DISORDERS

Irregular action of the bowels, failing appetite and biliousness frequently have their origin in some disorder of the liver. The importance of the liver can be understood when we consider even some of the functions it performs. It filters the blood and, in the process, neutralises any toxic substances in it, and does this at a rate of 1.7 litres (3 pints) every minute. It converts carbohydrates, proteins and fats so that they can be of use to the body. It makes bile, enzymes and proteins.

If you are simply feeling 'liverish', take an honest look at your intake of fast or fried foods, of fat and of course of alcohol.

An old remedy for liver disorders is the inner rind of the stalk and root of the barberry

(*Berberis vulgaris*). Macerate one teaspoonful to the litre (1¾ pints) in cold water for quarter of an hour and bring slowly to the boil; leave to infuse away from the heat for twenty minutes. Take a cupful morning and evening.

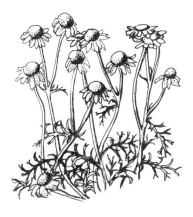

Camomile

Couch grass (*Agropyrum repens*) is another well-known remedy. For hundreds of years an infusion of the rhizome of couch grass was given in hospital to sufferers from some liver complaints. Put a handful of couchgrass leaves, chopped fine, in your salad every day for a while and you may find that you no longer feel 'liverish'. If you wish to save the rhizome for year-round use, gather it either in the spring or in the autumn, when its active principles are at their peak. Remove all minor rootlets and dry it in the sun, then chop it up and store it. Cats and dogs eat couch grass as a purge and butchers report that, while they find plenty of gallstones in cattle which they slaughter in the winter, they never find any in those slaughtered in spring and summer, when they have been eating couch grass.

The sapwood of the lime tree, i.e. the wood between the bark and the hard wood, taken as an infusion is an old French remedy for liver disorders. In matters affecting the liver, as in the case of the kidneys, the dandelion will be found to be your best friend; it is a balanced diuretic, replacing the potassium which is usually lost in diurectic action.

Mix aniseed, fennel, rosemary, mint, chervil, savory and basil in equal amounts. Infuse a cupful of this tea and take after meals as a liver tonic. An alternative tea is made from equal parts of dandelion and hops. Fennel, camomile and agrimony teas are also useful, or one made from the leaves of horseradish. Have a teaspoonful of apple cider vinegar in warm water several times a day. Eat artichokes and asparagus, beetroot, barley, cucumber cabbages and cauliflowers. Take fresh strawberries when possible and get kelp tablets from a health food shop. Apples, prunes, tomatoes and lemons will tone up the liver, as will barley water. See 'Kidney Diseases' on page 135.

MEMORY PROBLEMS

Much is said today about Alzheimer's disease causing lapses of memory, but there are very many other possible causes of this irksome complaint. The latest American research speculates that the onset of amnesia with the coming of old age is in most cases due to failure on the part of the sufferer to make a mental effort to remember. Then there are those who say that when your memory fails, blame overwork if you wish to believe yourself young, or simply amnesia if you admit to getting old.

Bad circulation of blood to the brain can cause memory loss. So can a poor diet. Elderly people who live alone frequently neglect themselves and do not eat properly. This deficiency is compounded by the diminishing ability of the body to absorb its required nourishment from food. As in many other aspects of bodily care, the cure sometimes seems a long way from the disease. If, for instance, an ageing friend complains of memory loss and you recommend a cup of sage tea to improve the appetite, or rosemary to stimulate the digestion and liver, you may be greeted with scepticism. But such are the mysteries of the body, and many are the apparently disconnected but actually appropriate remedies for ailments of all sorts. Who would be a doctor?

There are numerous aids to memory among the herbs. A wineglassful of rosemary infusion should be taken cold; if taken hot it will cause perspiration. The balm or lemon balm, taken as the rosemary is taken, is said to be the best possible remedy for failing memory. It was a favourite among university students in the days before coffee and cigarettes brought their doubtful assistance. A substance called choline is said to improve memory. You will get it in meat and vegetables and will make it yourself if your intakes of lecithin and B vitamins are adequate. But, over and above these remedies, treat your memory like a muscle and keep flexing it. When you make that effort it will repay you handsomely.

MIGRAINE

Many conditions involving headache get called 'migraine', but the real thing, to those who have suffered it, is unmistakable. The immediate cause of the excruciating pain involved is a swelling of the blood vessels in the head. Connections between migraine and the taking of certain foods have long been noticed by sufferers. Constipation will give you a savage headache and make a real migraine much worse. Chocolate, ice cream, cheese and red wine are notorious 'triggers' for migraine attacks, and there seems to be an hereditary factor. But psychological factors also rank high in the list of causes, and in this area one can alleviate if not eliminate the affliction altogether. I know someone who only needs to sit down calmly and let a subconscious problem float into the conscious mind and be dismissed as unworthy of causing a headache, for the migraine to vanish as quickly as it had come. It would be interesting to know if migraines are as common in the mystic, mind-over-matter East as they are in the frantic, hyperactive West.

Apart from the established value of certain conventional tonics, several herbal preparations have been known to relieve, even in some cases to cure, the condition. An infusion of rosemary, of vervain or of limeblossom will be of some assistance. So will an infusion of lavender, using stalks, leaves and flowers. Angelica in infusion is said to be marvellous, but don't exceed two cupfuls in a day or you may not sleep well. In various parts of Africa basil is given as a cure for migraine; the leaves are chewed to settle the nerves. Dab a cold infusion of marigold on the eyes and forehead for relief.

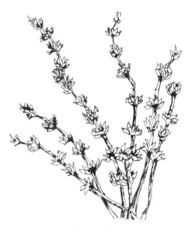

Lavender

Cabbage is probably the most accessible remedy for migraine. Wash the leaves well and pound them so that the juice comes to the surface, then warm them and apply to the area of the pain. Bind a few layers in place and renew them every few hours. An old folk medicine cure is to take a tablespoonful of honey internally and at the same time inhale the steam from equal parts of water and cider vinegar that has been boiled and allowed to cool slightly.

See also Feverfew on page 48.

NEURITIS/NEURALGIA

Generally speaking, neuritis or inflammation of the nerves results from trauma such as injury or strain. However, it can also betoken vitamin deficiency or a lack of calcium. In unusual cases it can be attributed to a virus.

The meadowsweet — in its most sophisticated manifestation, the aspirin — is taken for nerve pains of every kind, particularly for neuralgia, which is the form taken by nerve pains in the face. The latter often accompanies some dental problem; when it is rectified, the neuralgia diminishes or disappears altogether. The common ivy used externally can be most beneficial for nerve pains. The leaves are a sedative and have a regulatory effect on peripheral nerves. Chop them and apply directly to the skin. Alternatively make them into a poultice by mixing them in a ratio of one part of ivy leaf to two parts of bran in 250 ml (9 fl oz) of water. Warm for ten minutes, apply on a gauze pad and leave on the sore spot for an hour. One of the advantages of ivy is, of course, that it stays green all the year round. If you are picking ivy leaves in autumn look out for honey bees, especially after a bad summer. They will be frantically stocking up with ivy honey to carry them over the winter, and in a bad year this will make all the difference between survival and death for them.

A hot compress may also be used. Tarragon taken as an infusion is of considerable value in reducing the pain of neuralgia. Apply a decoction of vervain externally; the wild variety is far more valuable than the garden plant. A concentrated decoction of cranesbill (*Geranium robertanium*) — a dessertspoonful to 1 litre (1¾ pints) of water — can be applied externally to a facial neuralgia with satisfactory results. The rosemary was anciently used for nerve pains of various kinds, and if you apply a decoction to your face to cure neuralgia you may serve two purposes in one, as this is also a beauty treatment for removing freckles and ironing out wrinkles.

A cold infusion of tarragon taken after meals helps to relieve neuralgia.

Brush gently with a freshly picked stinging nettle arms and legs affected by neuritis. A tincture of St John's Wort also treats neuritis, as does bathing arms and legs in a decoction of yarrow.

Pick the flowers of thyme, mullein, yarrow and camomile. Put them in a bag and apply to the face for neuralgia; a tisane of all or any of these herbs can be taken at the same time.

RHEUMATISM

'Rheumatism' is really a catch-all word for a large variety of painful conditions involving swelling and general discomfort in soft tissues and muscles in various parts of the anatomy. It can have many causes and discussion continues as to the possible origins of some of its more unusual manifestations. It has been proposed that perverse emotional states such as resentment and even a puritanical kind of perfectionism may lie at the root of the condition. Given its complex and puzzling nature, it is obviously important to involve a competent practitioner in some relevant branch of medicine in the diagnosis and treatment of rheumatism. A professional herbalist will devote a great deal of time and thought to understanding the individual case and put together the kind of complex herbal remedy which space does not allow me to discuss here. However, a few observations on the kinds of food and herbs that have been found to help may be useful.

The simplest and some say most effective remedy for the rheumatic tendency is celery. Taken as part of a salad, or even as a tea (made with the crushed seeds), it has been found to have a remarkable effect in retarding the advance of the condition. Celery relieves pain and acts as a sedative, it aids digestion and encourages appetite and it is also antiseptic. Other herbs known to benefit the sufferer from rheumatism are red clover, yellow dock and yarrow. A cup of camomile tea has a soothing effect. When you have made the tea place the tea-bag on the affected joint; put it on cold if the joint is hot and warm if the joint is cold. Flowers of meadowsweet will ease painful joints, and an infusion of meadowsweet, taken three times daily, is beneficial. An infusion of blackcurrant leaves is an old remedy for rheumatism. An apple a day can help keep the rheumatism at bay. Eat it before breakfast or before going to bed to obtain maximum benefit. A decoction of powdered apple peel, drunk five times a day, is known to be of help, and so is the dandelion. A decoction of the dried root of parsley — indeed parsley in all its forms — will bring improvement.

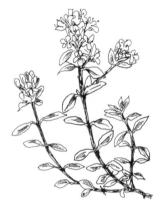

Thyme

Take frequent whole body baths which include two tablespoonfuls of Epsom salts. Compresses of comfrey should be applied externally, comfrey tea being taken internally at the same time. A cup of horsetail tea a day has a well-deserved reputation. Cook ramsons or wild garlic in milk, strain and drink the liquid once a day. Drink the tea of the stinging nettle and rub the affected parts with the fresh-picked stinging nettle (see 'Neuritis/Neuralgia'

on page 140). Rubbing the oil of wild thyme on the affected joints should bring relief. Lamb's-wool insoles should be worn in your shoes, at least during the winter. Allow for the thickness of the insole when you are purchasing new shoes or boots; otherwise you may get ingrowing toenails or corns to add to your misery. Bee stings are sometimes used (see 'Honey' on page 5). This rather drastic approach may not appeal to you so you will be heartened to know that honey contains some of the substance thought to give stings their power of healing.

RINGWORM

Ringworm is caused by a fungus. The name refers to the circular appearance of the patch of fungus on the skin, which can look like a worm but in fact has nothing to do with worms at all. It is sometimes contracted from handling farm animals, especially cattle, and this has given rise to a long litany of herbal treatments discovered by country people down the generations. The juice of borage made into a syrup is said to be good for the ringworm, both taken internally and rubbed on the sore place. A decoction of the tops of the hop plant applied externally is an old cure in places where the hops are grown. The common liverwort (*Hepatica*), taken in conjunction with sea bathing, was once thought helpful. Some people found that massaging the affected area with castor oil removed the fungus. Yarrow, mint, thyme and sage, infused in equal parts and with the addition of a decoction of crushed burdock root and drunk several times a day, is a fairly complicated herbal remedy for ringworm. A lotion of elder leaves with a little garlic and herb robert is also given for the complaint.

I cannot say how effective any of the above 'remedies' may be; doubtless there is some merit in each of them. But I can say that the ringworm gets more difficult to cure the longer it is present. I can also attest that I have often cured ringworm in friends by making a decoction of horsetail, to which I added a few drops of lavender, and applying it to the affected areas. As in all ailments of the skin, the approach should be hygienic. See that lint or any other fabric applied to the skin is clean and sterile. Try also to ensure that the remedy, having been applied, is not immediately rubbed off the skin by clothing. A clean bandage soaked in the decoction of

horsetail may be appropriate in some cases. A wetted (puce) copying pencil, drawn right around the ringworm, is a favourite folk cure in some country places. There is a fungicide in the lead reputed to destroy the 'worm'.

An old folk cure is an ointment made from lard and the tobacco ash from a pipe. Turpentine and bread soda mixed is also used. Repeated applications of cider vinegar are said to cure ringworm.

SINUSITIS

Your skull contains cavities called sinuses which communicate with your nostrils. These cavities sometimes become infected as a result of a cold or influenza. There are other possible reasons for infection which should not be overlooked, including a certain variety of tooth decay. The condition of sinusitis can become chronic and should always be taken seriously. There are many herbal preparations which treat and alleviate sinusitis, both directly and indirectly. By indirectly here I mean that any treatment for the general improvement of the mucous membrane must have a particular effect on the sinuses.

A decoction of the buds of

the Scots pine (*Pinus sylvestris*) is a remedy for sinusitis. Soak one tablespoonful in cold water for two hours. Heat and then boil for two minutes; leave to infuse for ten minutes. Take three cupfuls a day. This decoction can also be inhaled. Even walking through a pine forest will be found to have a most beneficial effect on the sinuses. Elderflowers will help to loosen catarrh. Yarrow tea will be very useful, as will peppermint tea. An infusion of eucalyptus leaves will help when inhaled; so will Olbas oil if it's mixed in hot water and inhaled. The wax removed by beekeepers from the cells of the honeycomb before the honey is extracted has its own natural antibiotic. This wax, or 'cappings' as it is called, should be chewed for as long as possible; it will do much to clear the sinuses. Swallow or spit out the wax according to taste. A clove of garlic kept in the mouth for an hour or two will achieve the same result, but don't bite the garlic or you'll burn your mouth.

There is one cause of acute sinusitis which leads to bleeding and the most horrible discharge through the mouth, and which for some reason often seems very hard to diagnose. The root of the second tooth from the back in either of the upper jaws sometimes penetrates one of the sinuses, and when this root rots, there are the above unhappy consequences. Nothing but the extraction of that tooth will solve the problem. Even if you have no pain, have the tooth properly X-rayed as a precaution. Your dentist will probably shriek with horror and do the rest. (I speak from experience.) A similar complaint in a dog can only be cured in the same way.

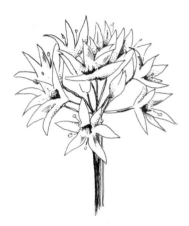

Ramsons (Wild Garlic)

Garlic taken in any of its shapes or forms can only benefit the sufferer from sinusitis. The fumes of garlic inhaled will help to kill the infection. White foods should be avoided like the plague; white bread and other white flour products, milk and milk products, white sugar and even potatoes all create mucus. If you go to a cheese and wine party, pass on the cheese and go easy on the wine. Inhale the steam from infused camomile. A compress of comfrey applied to the forehead and cheeks may bring some relief.

Much of what was discussed under 'Catarrh', page 112 and 'Common Colds and Chills', page 114 is applicable here.

SUNBURN

I found it ironic to be listening recently to a radio discussion on the ozone layer and the greenhouse effect while outside my window the annual May deluge was pouring cheerfully down in bucketfuls. The sun does sometimes shine in this part of the hemisphere, though, and apparently even when only trying to break through the clouds, it can have its dangers. The warnings about the holes in the ozone layer really have to be taken seriously, however great the temptation to smile through the rain.

Salt water and a seaside wind speed up the burning process. The virtual disappearance of the straw hat is showing up in the statistics. Fair-skinned and freckled people are extremely prone to skin cancer and the appalling fact that this disease can strike fifteen or twenty years after the fatal sun-bath is now well attested. So what do we do about the sun: sit inside waiting impatiently for it to shine, and then when it does, remember that it gives us skin cancer and remain indoors complaining about how heartless life can be? A bit of reason, as usual, goes a long way. Go into the sun, but be covered. Sunbathe at your peril; lying on the beach on a hot day under an umbrella can be a lot of fun.

Quince seeds which have been soaked for a few days form a healing lotion for sunburn. A weak infusion of either marigold or camomile, taken internally, can calm a distressed child (or adult) who has become feverish after being burnt. The fresh juice of the houseleek leaf has a soothing effect on burnt skin; so do cold sage tea, lemon juice, milk, or infusions of comfrey, camomile or elder allowed to cool.

Mix equal parts of cider vinegar and olive oil and if you have it handy add a dash of sesame oil. This will form an effective sun-blocking lotion for our usual northern summers. For stronger sunshine go for a commercial brand of sunblock. For skin which has been sunburnt use the same ingredients but increase the proportion of cider vinegar. Apply frequently and sip plenty of cool water.

If you are using calamine lotion to soothe sunburn, mix two teaspoonfuls of glycerine with equal parts of the lotion and carbonated spring water. Otherwise the skin may peel, particularly in the case of children, as calamine on its own tends to make the skin dry.

Any of the following will serve as an emergency lotion for sunburn: milk, cold Indian tea, cold sage tea, cold infusions of nettle, elderflower or comfrey. Dip freshly sliced cucumber in lemon juice and lay on the sunburnt skin. The juice of cucumber with a very little glycerine added has a fridge life of two to three days and will be effective for that period.

If you have been badly burnt see a doctor immediately.

ULCERS

Ulcers, both internal and external, are caused when tissues on the surface of the skin (or in the case of internal ulcers, the mucous membrane) break down. Acidic conditions inflame ulcers, but swallowing antacid tablets is not the solution. Most people have too little rather than too much acid in their systems — this applies to ulcer sufferers as much as to anyone else — and therefore taking antacid tablets and thereby reducing further the amount of acid in the system is very often only making the condition worse. The problem really arises because the symptoms of having too much acid in the stomach are exactly the same as the symptoms of having too little.

The professional herbalist will take a careful note of your symptoms and general health history, including signs of anxiety in your temperamental make-up, for an internal ulcer is one of the diseases frequently associated with anxious personalities. A great deal can be done to control temperamental tendencies if the patient is willing to learn how to 'talk himself down' in conditions of stress or even potential stress. But remember that a busy medical profession is geared more to prescribing cures than to taking the time to teach people methods of controlling their mental and emotional reactions. A visit to a yoga centre or enrolment in a transcendental meditation class could have a critical influence in helping you to recover from an ulcer.

Golden seal, available in

tablet form, can have a benign effect on the sufferer from internal ulcers. The best of all natural restorers of the mucous membrane is the blackberry. If you are making jam from the berries, keep the sugar to a minimum. That way you will both get the true flavour of this marvellous fruit and do the greatest good possible for your ulcer. A decoction of the leaves will be beneficial to your entire digestive tract. Drink clear carrot soup hot with meals. Comfrey, taken in any of its forms, heals the mucous membrane; macerate one tablespoonful of the chopped root for three hours and drink the resulting liquid several times each day.

Leg ulcers may benefit from a poultice of comfrey leaf, yarrow or marigold. However, the underlying condition that needs to be addressed is the presence of impurities in the blood. Again, the dandelion can come to the rescue, as well as the nettle (take the latter sparingly as over-indulgence could lead to a skin rash). A poultice made from sugar soaked in a decoction of walnut leaves is sometimes helpful with a particularly stubborn leg ulcer. A poultice of dock leaves or of cabbage leaves can also bring a measure of success. Remove the hard central vein from the leaves, shred the rest and apply with a bandage. Coal tar or Jeyes' Fluid were old remedies for leg ulcers, perhaps included in small proportions in comfrey ointment.

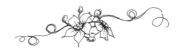